WORKOUTS THAT WORK
FOR WOMEN WHO WORK

WORKOUTS THAT WORK FOR WOMEN WHO WORK

Barbara Pearlman

Photographs by Kevin Lein

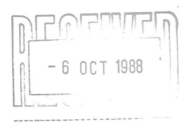
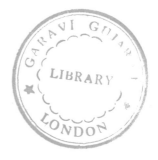

Arlington Books
King St, St James's
London

WORKOUTS THAT WORK
FOR WOMEN WHO WORK

First published in Great Britain 1988 by
Arlington Books (Publishers) Ltd
15–17 King St, St James's
London SW1

British Library Cataloguing-in-Publications Data

Pearlman, Barbara
Workouts that work for women who work
1.   Women. Physical fitness. Exercises
I.   Title
613.7'1'088042

ISBN 0–85140–742–0

Printed and bound in Great Britain by
The Hollen Press,
Slough.

Dedicated with admiration
to a dozen working women:
Miriam, Roz, Ciba, Lynn, Leslie, Wendy,
Sandi, Shirley, Bobbie, Ann, Ellen, and Lenore

CONTENTS

ACKNOWLEDGMENTS

I'm grateful to many who contributed and guided me in shaping this book. My thanks to my agent, Jane Dystel. To Lisa Wager for launching this book and to my editor, Casey Fuetsch. My gratitude to Alex Gotfryd for his valued assistance. I wish to thank Kevin Lein for his discerning eye and Cheryl Marks for her creative approach to hair and makeup. To all my students and private clients, thank you for making my work so rewarding. Affectionate gratitude to my family for giving me loving support as well as the time and space to write. A very special thanks to my son, Aaron, for his sensitivity and compassion and to my husband, Stephen, who has always encouraged me to stretch.

The bookstore shelves are bulging with exercise how-to's designed to shape up everyone from the pediatric set to the geriatric. Fast fixes to firm the bottom and flatten the stomach abound, and just about every Hollywood star has had a crack at shaping the inner thighs of American women. Yet, no exercise book has been written for the working woman that specifically focuses on two of her major concerns: (1) her limited time to exercise (2) the figure/posture problems that evolve from, or are aggravated by the nature of her work. This book presents effective, realistic solutions to those concerns.

Section I offers a series of short exercise routines that overcome inertia, resistance and all excuses not to exercise. You will be able to slip these simple regimens into your hectic schedule almost effortlessly, before or after work, while at home or at the office, wearing anything from a business suit to a nightie. These pint-sized segments can be mixed and matched or gathered together into a tuning up, toning down workout. Above all, they truly deliver results while respecting your limited time and oftentimes limited space.

I encourage you to "exercise your options" by choosing from a varied selection of mini routines. Depending on your needs as well as your time restrictions on a particular day, you can practice one, several or all

INTRODUCTION

of them. Or, by linking several segments together, you can, if you wish, extend the time you devote to your daily workout. And, because of the choices presented, you will be spared the boredom that invariably results from repeating the same exercise routine day after day.

Section II of the book presents four programmes designed to combat the effects of your job. These routines zero in on correcting or eliminating the body-related problems resulting from your particular profession. Naturally, I encourage you to practice more than one routine if your needs are multiple. For instance, if your job requires you to be on your feet all day and you tend to stand slumped and round-shouldered, it would be both advantageous and advisable for you to concentrate your efforts on the routines in chapters 8 and 9. The individual routines can be practiced in their entirety, or you can select several exercises from each, combining the movements in an endless variety of personally designed segments.

As a fitness consultant to working women of all shapes, sizes, ages and occupations, I have welcomed their valuable sentiments and suggestions. Client input has guided me in my work over the past fifteen years as well as in the development of this book's format. Most working women agree they are more apt to follow an exercise programme faithfully if it is manageable and, above all, not too time-consuming. When her fitness demands are excessive (or unrealistic), the average working woman becomes an exercise dropout. So too, working women concur that the nature of their job affects not only the appearance of their figures but the condition of their bodies as well.

In formulating and writing this book, considerable time was devoted to interviewing women in varying jobs and professions . . . from the patent lawyer to the air stewardess, the seamstress to the songwriter. In addition, I used my office/studio as a "research lab," with client assistance, to create the best and most effective routines possible. The programme that evolved offers variety and flexibility (so you won't become bored), yet it's easy enough to follow so you won't have trouble sticking with it.

The exercises blend several movement techniques including dance-exercise stretches, modified yoga postures and effective orthopaedic movements for strengthening the back and perfecting posture. I do not want to suggest, however, that this programme addresses *all* your fitness needs. A regular aerobic activity should be included in your personal fitness plan as well. Aerobic exercises are those that commit you to consume more oxygen and are essential for cardiovascular fitness. For aerobic exercise to be effective, your goal should be to get your heart beating at the target pulse rate for twenty to thirty minutes. Your target pulse rate tells you just how strenuous your workouts should be. The target rate should be from 70 to 85 percent of your maximum pulse rate, which you can estimate by subtracting your age from 220.

Sound complicated? It's not. Let's suppose that a thirty-five-year-old woman wants to know how hard she should exercise. Her first step is to establish her maximum pulse rate, which is 185 (220 minus 35). Her target pulse rate (70 percent to 85 percent of 185) ranges from 130 to 157. If her exercise program is vigorous enough to keep her heart beating within this range for twenty to thirty minutes, four times a week, she's getting aerobic benefits from her workout. If it's not, she's not becoming aerobically fit. Above all, it is important that you choose an aerobic activity, be it a sport (e.g., cycling, swimming, jogging) or rhythmic movement (such as dancing) that appeals to you and can be woven into the fabric of your days with both ease and pleasure.

In order to maximize mileage from these workouts, anywhere, any-time, in any clothes, it's essential that you master some very fundamental exercise principles.

Concentrate and involve yourself as you move. Be aware of the various parts of your body that are moving with each exercise, no matter how simple it may be. Try to develop a sense of the total involvement of all parts of your body, even though the action may be concentrated on one or two specific areas. Understand which muscles control which movements. This will not only help you to perform the exercises correctly, but it will also increase and improve your overall balance and coordination.

Never strain. You need not *agonize* to exercise. Every woman should learn the difference in *her* body between pain and the feel of a muscle being worked. Pain is always a red light that something is wrong. You and only you are the best judge of how far to go and how long to continue. Always keep in mind that when any part of your body is genuinely uncomfortable, it is an indication that you're applying yourself too strenuously. Let up a bit.

Keep your abdominals contracted. As you exercise, whether standing, sitting or doing floor work, constantly remind yourself to pull in your abdomen (without holding your breath). Keeping your abdominal muscles contracted applies when you're concentrating your efforts on your other muscle groups as well. In my opinion, it's really the key to moving with proper alignment. Once you perfect the "tuck" and can work with abdominal control, all movements become more effective.

Remember to breathe. Correct breath control is essential in order to keep your muscles well oxygenated. Oftentimes, particularly when one is new to exercise, the tendency is to hold one's breath or to breathe in a shallow manner. Constricting your breath during exertion can cause light-headedness or a dull headache. When you're first learning an exercise, simply relax and breathe as naturally as possible. Then, once you're familiar with the movement, pay close attention to proper breath control. Always exhale through your mouth (as if blowing out a candle) on the exertion and inhale through your nose (nasal passages warm, dampen and clean the air before it enters the lungs) on the release. I find that emphasizing the exhalation, in particular, works best for most students, since inhalation tends to come more naturally. That is why, in many cases, I simply note the timing for the breathing out. The exhalation is above all important when you are using weights of any kind. Be certain it always accompanies the exertion (i.e., lift).

Never sacrifice good placement for speed. It is far more important to execute an exercise correctly than rapidly. If time is limited and you are unable to complete an entire sequence of movements, don't pressure yourself in order to do so. Choose only what you are able to manage with precision and care.

Avoid jerky, bouncing motions. Sharp, staccato movements can place harmful demands on your joints and muscles. Bouncing can tear the web of connective tissue that holds muscles together. This is not only painful in itself but causes fluid to enter the muscle, producing the tight or slightly swollen sensation you experience the day after you exercise too zealously. No matter which movements you're doing—the supersimple or tougher toners—always move with as much fluidity and grace as possible. Instead of a bounce, think in terms of a more gentle, pulsing motion.

Finally, while practicing the exercises, try to avoid common movement errors such as hyperextending your elbows and knees, overarching your back, tensing your neck and shoulders and swinging your limbs with abandon. All of these errors detract from the effectiveness of an exercise and place harmful and excessive demands on your body instrument.

Do not become discouraged if you cannot duplicate the positions demonstrated in the photographs. They are presented as goals to be worked towards rather than what should be copied immediately. So too, if the instructions call for repeating the movement twenty times and you find the number excessive, build up to it gradually.

Be prepared to experience some minimal soreness if you have not been exercising. Your muscles are being used in unaccustomed ways. Lazy, inactive muscles are naturally going to protest somewhat. This is absolutely normal and should not cause you any concern. As the days progress, providing you incorporate some regular exercise, you will notice that the minor aches you formerly experienced will disappear.

Please give adequate emphasis to the release exercises I often recommend that you do between sets. Movements such as knee hugs or slow head rolls serve to relax muscle tension and should not be omitted.

Regardless of your age or shape, however, if you have had any serious medical problem or have been inactive for a significant length of time, it is always advisable to consult with your physician before attempting any new exercise programme.

Above all, no matter how crammed and crunched your days might be, taking time out for movement is essential. Promise yourself you'll do some exercise daily. Even several minutes can be a worthwhile investment. A few energizing in-bed stretches can lure your body toward mobility and start your day on the right foot. Simple Relaxercises will help you manage your stress rather than having it manage you. Remember too, you don't have to be in leotards to be fit; the benefits of exercise are on a continuum. Exercise stretches your day by giving you the stamina to accomplish more. As a working woman juggling combined professional and personal responsibilities, you owe it to yourself to feel and look your best. By making movement an important and integral ingredient in your life, you will improve not only your look, but your *outlook* as well.

SECTION

I

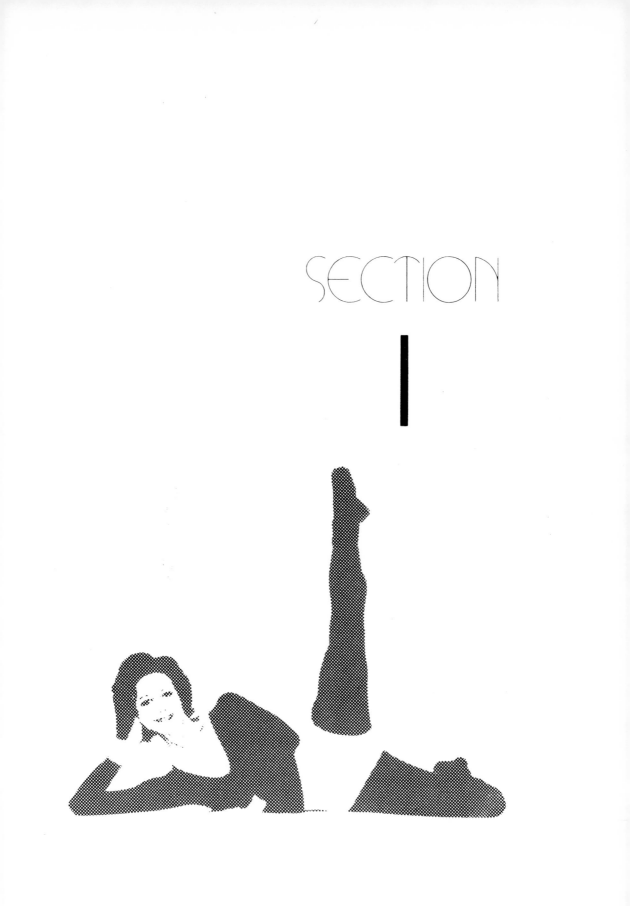

T here aren't enough hours in the day" is the sentiment shared by most working women. And getting enough sleep to face your days with a minimum of wear and tear becomes a challenge in itself.

There are two distinct kinds of tiredness. One results after physical activity. For me, this fatigue feels quite pleasant and generally means that I'm going to fall asleep with little effort. The second kind of tiredness is not as readily welcomed. This is a mental and emotional fatigue that usually follows a day of stress, tension and worry. It's often characterized by an unpleasant feeling of irritability, anger and, for many working women, that sense of just feeling *overwhelmed.* Many of my clients express concern about the physical manifestations that accompany this sort of fatigue . . . tensed muscles, stomach spasms and headaches. You don't fall asleep easily from this kind of weariness. Generally you lie in bed worrying, tense, too tired to sleep.

Frequently, by just doing some simple relaxation exercises, you can establish a sense of calm that will set the stage for sleep. Some of my favourites are the dangle and the knee hug. They sure beat becoming hostage to sleeping pills or other nighttime tranquilizing drugs.

You and you alone know how much sleep you need in order to function at your

1

IN-BED STRETCHES

best. We obviously differ in the amount of sleep we require. So too, there are "night people" who seem to perk up after dark and "day people" who begin to yawn as early as 9 P.M. (It appears that the owls rarely change into larks or vice versa.) Some women can get along on as little as five hours' sleep and others are veritable zombies with anything less than nine. I personally require about seven. Granted, I can manage on less, but not for too many days in succession. It finally catches up with me and then I am unable to face professional and family responsibilities with a clear head. Knowing your own body and what it requires, be it food, exercise or sleep is essential to every working woman's well-being.

Remember too, during sleep the largest organ of your body, your skin, appears to rest as well. That's why the term "beauty sleep" isn't a misnomer. It's a phrase that means exactly what it states. Your looks truly do improve with sleep and can certainly suffer when you're lacking it in large doses, the reason being that sleep is essential to the skin-making process. Skin cells divide and make new cells twice as fast while you sleep.

Think how luxurious one long, indulgent all-over stretch feels in the morning. Now imagine how much better a few specially targeted body stretches could make you feel. It's unrealistic to expect your body to spring into action with the buzz of your alarm clock. Instead, take a tip from an awakening cat and S-T-R-E-T-C-H in every which way. Begin your day with some or all of the in-bed exercises that have been included in this section. Simply roll over and do them right on top of the mattress. Although I have included suggested repetitions for each exercise, the best criterion for how many is what feels good to you. Take them easy, take them slowly. But do take them seriously, since they can truly make the difference as to how your day gets launched. Remember, waking up need not be a head-on collision with gravity.

1

Rubber-band Stretch

1. Lie on your back, legs extended. Relax your arms at your sides.

2. Inhale deeply, stretching your left arm overhead as you simultaneously flex your left foot. Feel the stretch from your fingertips to your heel. Hold for 2 counts. Lower your arm and relax your foot as you exhale. Repeat on the right side.

Repetition: Three times on each side

(Tip) Poor sleep posture is a sure invitation to backaches. Avoid lying on your stomach, a position that increases the spine lumbar curve. Best bet: lie on your side with your hips and knees slightly bent.

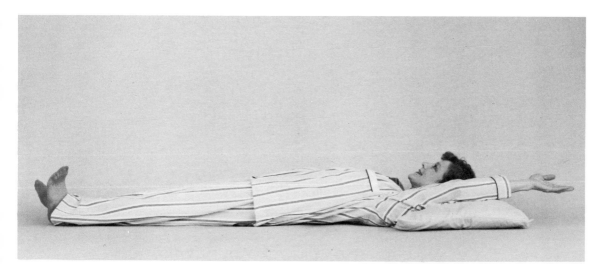

2

Hamstring Stretch

1. Lie on your back with your left knee bent and the foot resting on the bed. Extend your right leg up, toes pointed. Clasp your hands behind your knee.

2. Gently ease your leg towards your body, trying to keep it as straight as possible. Repeat 6 times with the foot pointed, then with it flexed. Repeat on the left leg.

Repetition: One complete set on each leg

(Tip) To be effective, naps should be limited to a half hour or forty-five minutes. That way you pass through early stages of restorative sleep, but never reach the deep sleep that can be disruptive if interrupted.

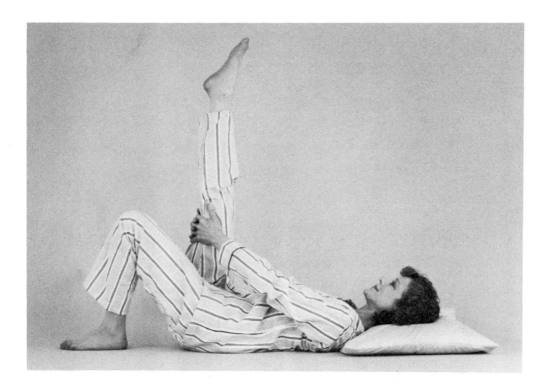

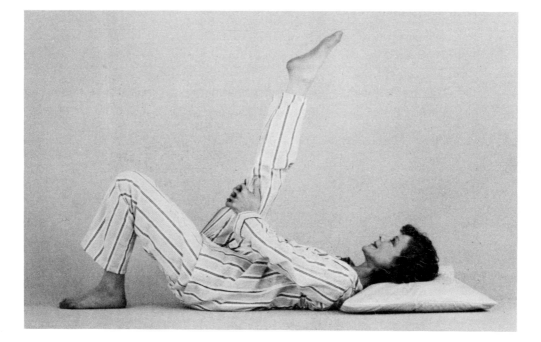

3

Roll Over

1. Lie on your back with your left leg extended. Interlace your fingers and place your hands behind your head. Cross your right foot over your left leg and rest it on the bed near your thigh.

2. Keeping your right shoulder stationary, lower the knee as far to the left as you can. Hold the stretch for 6 counts, breathing naturally. Then repeat with the left knee.

Repetition: Twice on each side

This stretch can be soothing if you have sciatic problems affecting the lower back. It's a wonderful relaxation exercise as well.

(Tip) Treated well, a good innerspring mattress will usually last about ten years.

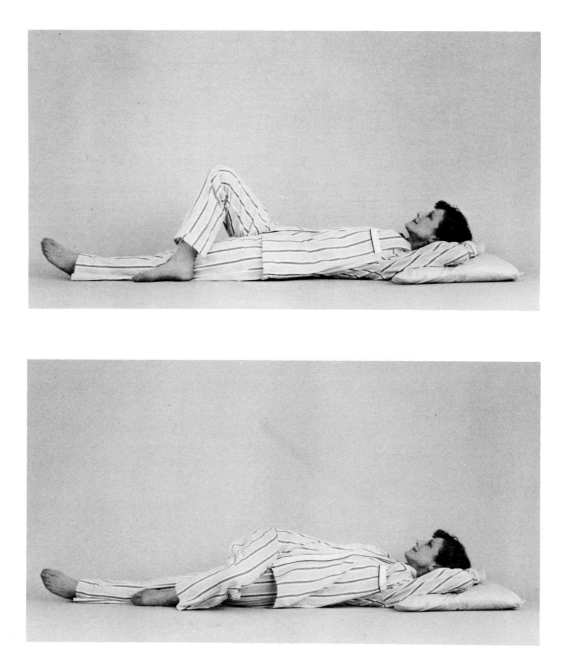

4

Knee Rock

1. Lie on your back with your knees bent toward your body. Interlace your fingers and place them below your knees.

2. Rock your knees in a gentle back-and-forth movement.

Repetition: Ten times

This is also effective as a relaxer between sets of challenging abdominal work.

(Tip) To test a mattress, lie on it, noting whether it pushes firmly, but with resilience, against your hips and shoulders.

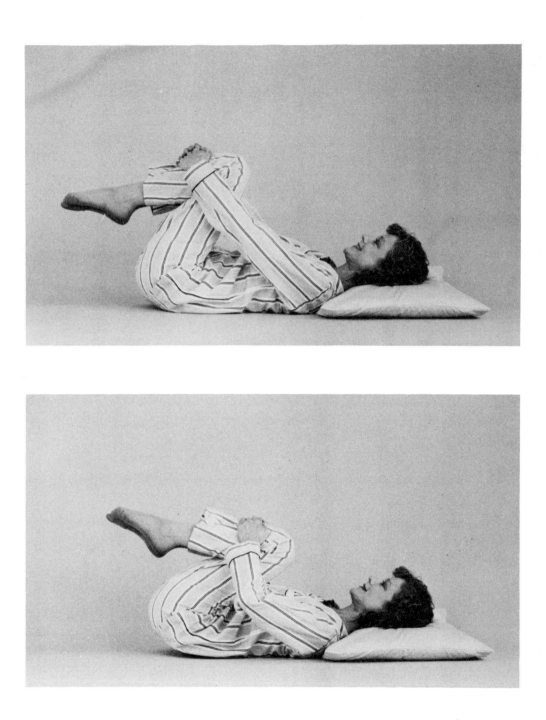

5

Double Leg Lift

1. Lie on your back with your knees bent close to your chest. Place your hands behind your head.

2. Extend both legs up as you exhale and tighten your abdominals. Lower your legs to the original position.

Repetition: Ten times

(Tip) Cramps, the S.O.S. of muscles in distress, are a body clue that is anything but subtle. When you're jolted awake by a calf cramp, gently flex your foot upward to stretch it against the cramped muscle for relief. Gentle kneading massage can help as well.

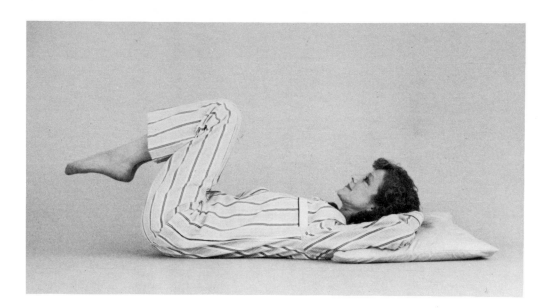

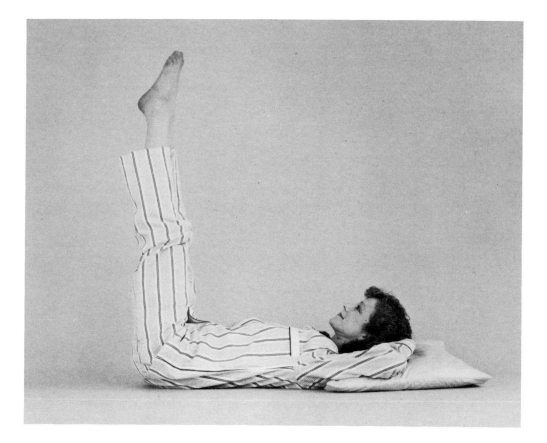

6

Upper Body Stretch

1. Sit with your knees bent, feet parallel and hip-width apart. Interlace your hands behind your body.

2. Lower your head and round your back as you simultaneously lift your arms. Hold for 2 counts.

Then lower your arms and straighten your back to the original position. Exhale on the lowering motion and inhale on the lift.

Repetition: Four times

(Tip) The best way to anchor regular sleep is to get up at the same time, no matter when you go to bed.

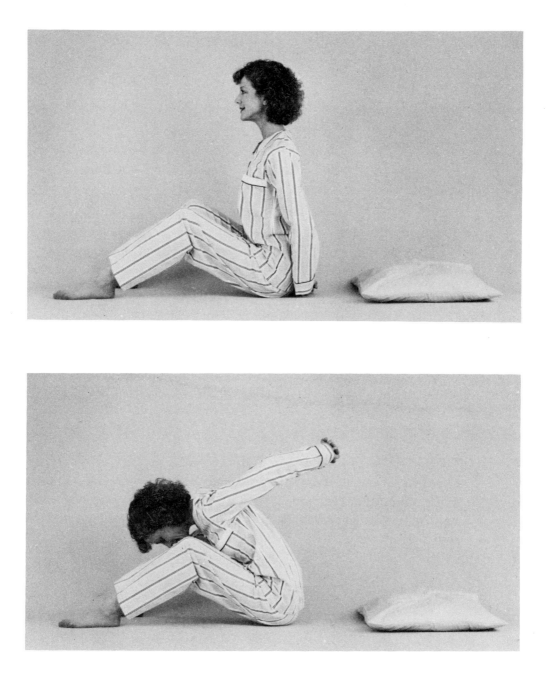

7

Palms Up Stretch

1. Sit with your ankles crossed. Rest your interlaced hands behind your head, elbows wide apart.

2. Extend your arms up, palms facing the ceiling. Lower them to the original position. Exhale on the extension and inhale on the release.

Repetition: Eight times

This exercise should awaken those sleepy upper-back muscles. It's also an effective exercise to combat round shoulders.

(Tip) Does your pillow droop like a deflated balloon when you support it over your outstretched arm? If so, it's probably time to invest in a new one. A good pillow cradles the neck so that your head is aligned with the rest of your body.

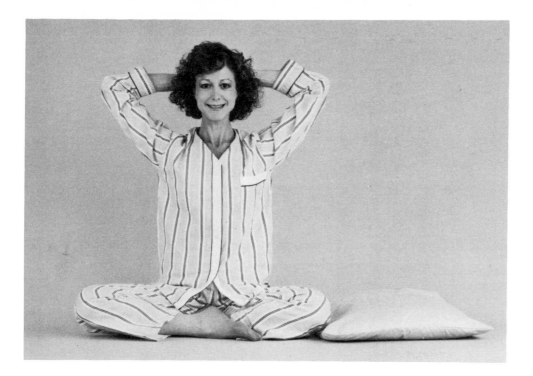

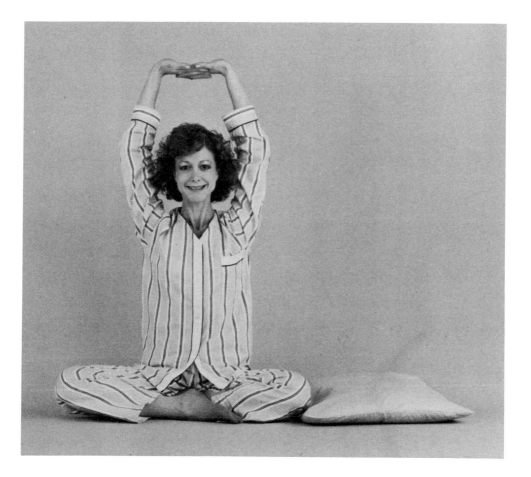

2

A.M. AWAKENER

For the majority of working women, mornings can be the most frenetic time of day . . . particularly if the demands of your household are numerous. Preparing breakfast, tending to domestic chores and organizing yourself for the workday ahead can leave you close to exhaustion before you even leave the house.

Many of my clients prefer to shave off some sleep time in order to get their exercise "out of the way" and "over with" prior to work. Others claim their body clock simply can't cope with the idea of bolting out of bed for buttock lifts or a sunrise jog. So, if pressuring yourself to exercise adds yet another stress to your morning, believe me, it's not worth it.

On mornings when you're unable to manage anything more than the in-bed stretches, that's perfectly fine. If, however, you have a few additional minutes (and your body and psyche agree), try some or all of the exercises that have been included in the A.M. Awakener. The purpose of this segment is simply to activate your circulation and prompt a healthy good-morning flush. The entire routine should take approximately eight minutes from start to finish.

Remember, too, this regimen can serve as the preface to the P.M. Pickup. By combining the two, you will derive an energizing, figure-firming workout.

Since you will be shifting still drowsy muscles (and mood) into a higher gear, begin by stretching slowly and with care. Make certain your movements are as fluid as possible and that you place proper emphasis on correct breathing technique. As for the brief prancing-in-place segment, since you will probably be still in your sleepwear and barefoot, it's important that you refrain from lifting your feet off the floor. That's particularly important to keep in mind if your bedroom floor is not well padded. Simply raise your heels and move your arms continuously. By so doing, you will activate your circulation and experience the refreshing effect of this A.M. segment.

A.M. AWAKENER

1

Prance in Place

1. Prance in place lifting only your heels. Keep the balls of your feet in contact with the floor. Each time your right heel lifts, stretch your arms forward. As your left heel lifts, pull your elbows back. Try to move your arms rhythmically in time with the footwork, keeping your breathing smooth and steady. Continue the prancing motion for one minute to activate your blood flow.

(Tip) If you rely on cartoned orange or grapefruit juice for your morning dose of C, transfer the juice to an airtight container after opening. Vitamin C breaks down the minute it's exposed to air. If it is left in an open carton for a couple of days, its health powers can dwindle to zero.

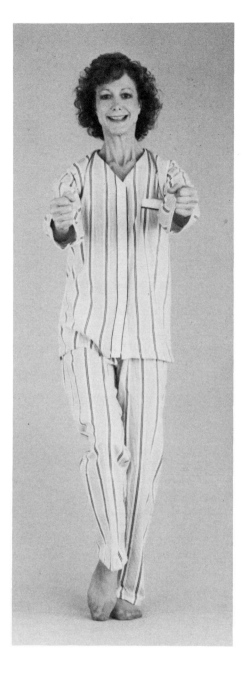

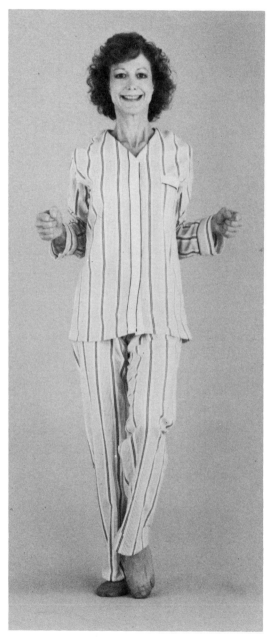

2

Swing Through

1. Stand with your feet parallel and about shoulder-width apart. Extend your arms overhead.

2. Lower your head and round your back as you bend your knees and gently, without forcing the movement, swing your arms be-tween your legs. Swing forward and lift to the original position, making certain you lengthen your spine and inhale with each lift.

Repetition: Ten times

(**Tip**) Your personal "prime time" is the pivot for planning your day. When do you feel most alert, most capable of clear, concentrated thinking? When possible, schedule priority tasks during your peak time in order to be most productive.

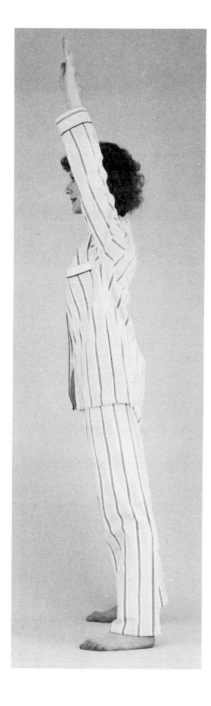

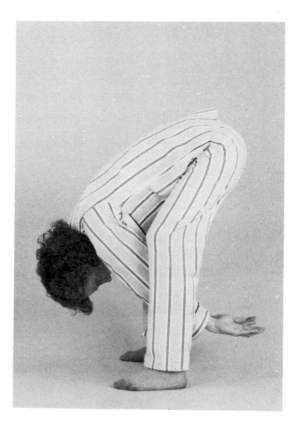

3

Tilt

1. Stand with your feet wide apart and slightly turned out. Interlace your hands overhead, palms facing up.

2. Tilt from side to side, keeping your hips stationary and your knees slightly bent. Lengthen your spine on the center lift for a good torso stretch. Exhale on the tilt and inhale on the lift.

Repetition: Six times to each side

(**Tip**) Eat more cereals and breads at breakfast . . . less fat. These carbohydrates are not only a heart-healthy choice, but also a preferred energy source for your muscles.

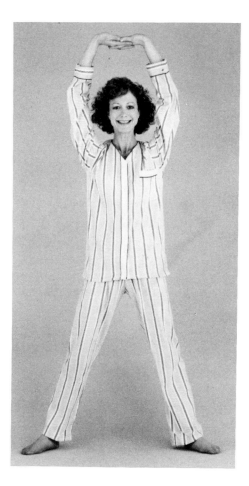

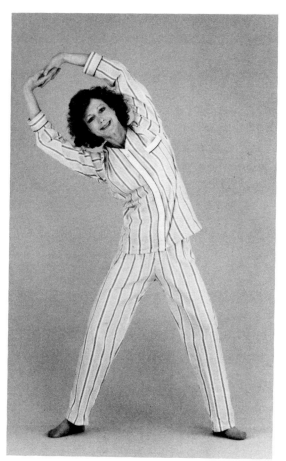

4

Foot Touch Lunge

1. Stand with your feet wide apart and slightly turned out.

2. Lunge to the right, trying to touch your left hand to your right foot. Let your right arm swing and lift behind your body. Then lunge to the left. Try to keep the leg that is not bending as straight as possible and your breathing relaxed.

Repetition: Six times to each side

(Tip) Avoid peak-hour delays. Make appointments with home-repair people, doctors, etc., for a time when you can be first on the list.

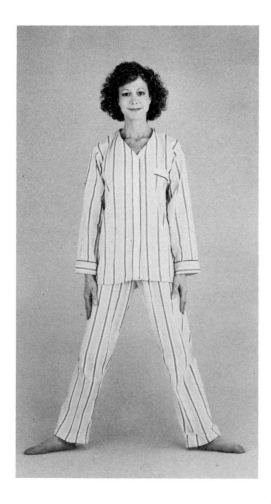

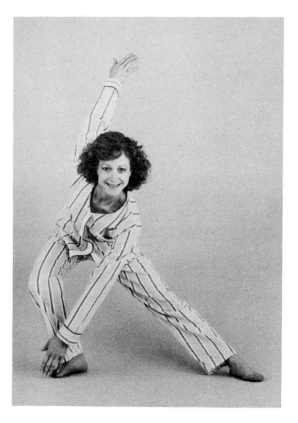

5

Overhead Stretch

1. Stand with your feet shoulder-width apart and slightly turned out. Extend your arms overhead.

2. Stretch upward, first with your right arm, then with your left. Imagine climbing higher and higher on a rope. Feel the lift in your rib cage, breath steady and relaxed.

Repetition: Six times on each side

(Tip) Skipping breakfast can sabotage a weight-reduction diet by causing a drastic dip in your blood-sugar level, signalling your body to add fuel, *fast*.

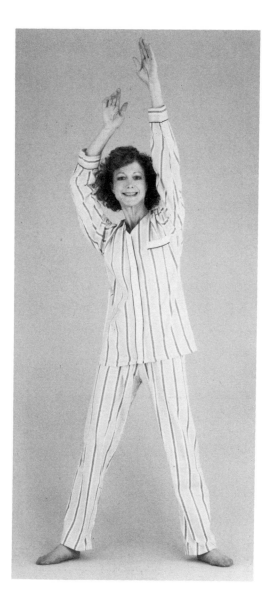

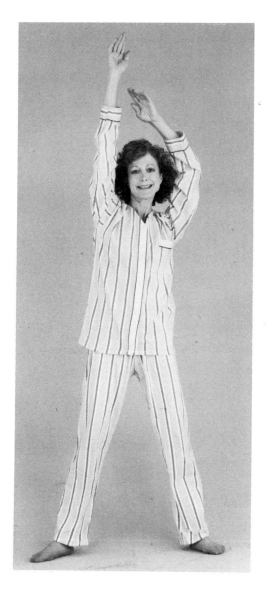

6

Plié

1. Stand with your feet shoulder-width apart and slightly turned out. Extend your arms overhead, crossing them at the wrists.

2. Bend your knees as you simultaneously lower your arms out to the sides until your wrists cross low, in front of your body. Then straighten your legs as you lift your arms out to the sides until your wrists cross overhead. Inhale on the upward stretch.

Repetition: Twelve times

With any plié movement, try to bend your knees directly over your feet, keeping your shoulders in line with your hips. Buttocks tucked under, abdomen in.

(**Tip**) The best time of the month for breast self examination: about one week after your period, when your breasts are usually not tender or swollen. After menopause, check breasts on the first day of each month.

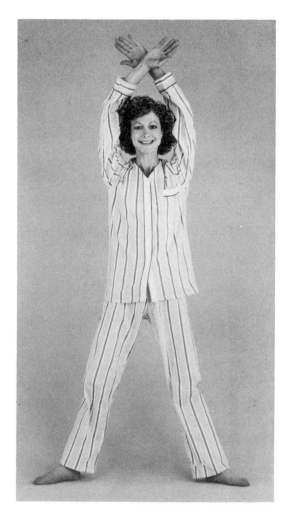

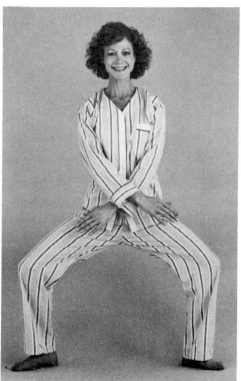

3

SHOWER SHAPERS, BATH AND TOWEL TONERS

Is there anything more relaxing than submerging yourself in a bath of warm, herb-scented water and just lying there, listening to the tiny whisper of soap bubbles? There may be, but to my knowledge, it has yet to be invented. If you're like me, most of the time all you can do is pop in and out of the bath, settling for a quick once-over sudsing. But when you have time to spare, and a chance to recharge your batteries, pamper your body and soothe your stressed-out psyche by soaking in the bath.

The waters of the bath can truly be restorative after a hectic, nonstop workday. So too, bath time can set the scene for the transition between day and night, work and home, solitude and socializing. But most of all, bathing is yet another way to make an "appointment" with yourself . . . to take time out for *you.* Time out to treat yourself kindly, at home or on the road.

Without detracting from the essential enjoyment of this experience, I've included in this section a few gentle stretches that will enhance the benefits of your bath and shower. You may wish to create some of your own as well. Just as the steamy heat from bath water urges pores open, making them more receptive to skin softeners and cleansers, heat and humidity relax muscles, increasing their stretch-and-contract capabilities.

You don't need an oversize bath in which to perform the bath toners; a standard one will do. The magic ingredient is water. The more there is in the bath, the more demanding any exercise becomes, because of the resistance element. Your bath water should not be too hot, which is drying for the skin as well as enervating to the body. Perform any bath exercise at a leisurely pace, never forcing the movements. And please remember, a nonskid mat is a *must* for either the bath or shower shapers.

Personally, I prefer to shower in the morning (it's the only way I can really wake up) and save my leisure soaks for the evening. It becomes my getaway time from the world . . . from business calls, household demands and family uprisings. Frequently, I follow my evening bath stretches with a few mind-calming relaxation exercises. Combining the two creates a very effective duo, one that many of my clients welcome prior to bedtime. Should you prefer, however, these or any bath exercises can be done in the morning. Practising them in conjunction with the A.M. Awakener makes for a pleasant and effective morning routine.

If your preference is to shower instead, it's yet another opportunity to almost effortlessly weave a few stretches into your morning shape-up routine. Warm shower water can be truly therapeutic for diminishing early-morning stiffness. At night, these shower shapers can help dissolve a day's tension in almost no time at all. When I do any stretching in the shower, I generally begin by directing the water to my upper back, then I change the direction for a lower back massage. Again, a nonskid surface is imperative.

When time permits, try to do a few minutes of warm-ups while your bath water is running. I use my towel rack or the sink ledge as a support when doing simple knee bends or standing push-ups. Once you're ready for toweling off, blot (never rub) yourself dry and, before placing the towel back on the rack, take a minute for a towel toner.

With this short and simple three-part routine, you can turn your bathroom into your own private spa. This regimen is practical, since you can do it just about anywhere you go. Your exercise spirit need not dampen simply because of the somewhat cramped quarters of a bathroom.

BATH TONERS

1

Tightening Tuck

1. Sit with your heels raised, toes pointed and resting on the bottom of the bath. Use your hands for additional support.

2. Contract your buttock and abdominal muscles. Hold for 3 slow counts, then relax. Make certain that you exhale (through your mouth) as you contract, in order not to strain unnecessarily.

Repetition: Six times

(Tip) A loofah, the dry, rough-textured gourd that swells and softens when wet, is effective for sloughing off dead skin, particularly on the bottoms of tired, overworked feet.

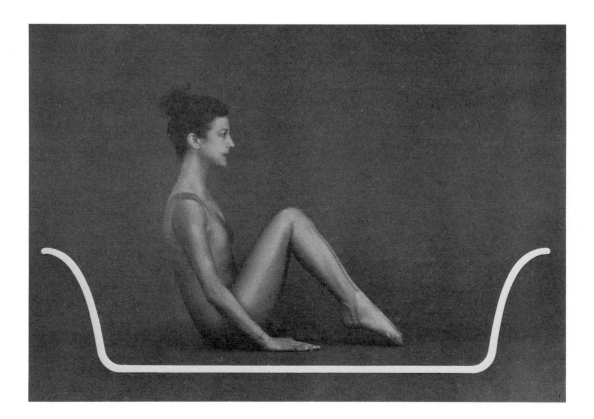

2

Leg Circle

1. Sit with your left knee bent and your hands clasped below it. Extend your right leg in front, foot flexed and turned out.

2. Keeping the right foot raised and turned out, form an outward circle with it 12 times, making certain your abdominals remain contracted. Lower the leg and repeat on the left leg.

Repetition: Three sets on each leg

These circles tighten the inner thigh. As an alternative for the front of the thigh, you can also do leg lifts with the foot flexed and the heel down.

(Tip) Bath basics: Water should be 90–98 degrees F. To relieve tired, aching muscles, go slightly warmer. Twenty minutes is the ideal soaking time. Any longer tends to dry the skin.

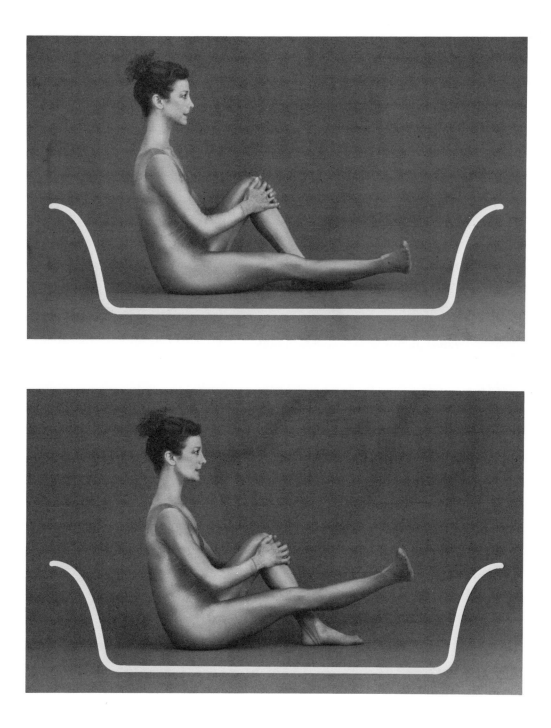

3

Elbow Squeeze

1. Sit with your knees bent, feet parallel and shoulder-width apart. Place your right hand on the tub floor. Bend your left arm and place your elbow against your left inner thigh and your palm against your right knee.

2. Press your legs toward each other as firmly as possible. Hold this maximal contraction for 6 counts. Do not hold your breath. Repeat with the other arm resisting the press.

Repetition: Three times with each arm

This seemingly easy exercise really zeros in on the inner thigh.

(Tip) Mix a cup of milk, a capful of bath oil and swirl it into your bath. Milk has substantial soothing properties and the mixture is a truly effective emollient.

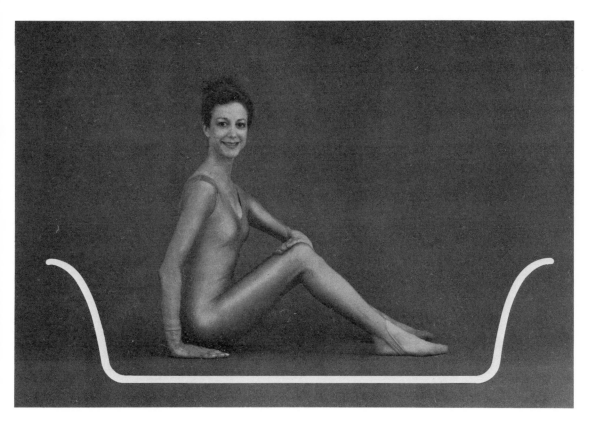

SHOWER SHAPERS

1

Head Tilt

1. Stand with your feet apart. Relax your arms at your sides.

2. Gently tilt your head back, feeling a comfortable stretch in your neck. Next drop your head forward, lowering your chin. Take your time, allowing the shower to massage the nape of your neck.

Repetition: Six complete sets

In addition to the tilt, include slow head rotations as well as shoulder shrugs and rolls as part of your shower routine.

(Tip) Showers can help to alleviate backaches and pains. Sit on the floor of the bath, resting your head on your knees. Let the warm water pour down your back, shoulders and the nape of your neck. Two minutes can really make a difference.

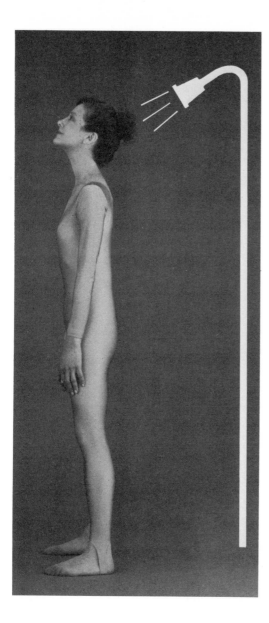

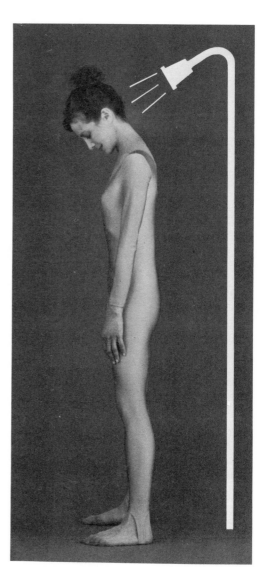

2

Parallel Feet Pulse

1. Stand with your feet parallel and shoulder-width apart. Relax your arms at your sides.

2. Bend your knees over your toes, keeping your shoulders in line with your hips. In this lowered position, gently pulse downward 4 times. Straighten your knees, and repeat the sequence.

Repetition: Four sets

A plié practiced with your feet parallel, instead of turned out, will strengthen the front of your thighs (the quadriceps).

(Tip) For the silkiest shave, timing is everything. Shave your legs about three minutes into a shower or bath. At that point, hair is soaked and softened. Wait too long (more than fifteen minutes) to shave and skin swells slightly from having absorbed water. The slight puffiness makes getting close to hair follicles more difficult, so your shave won't be as close.

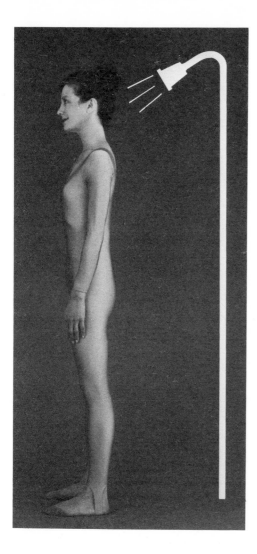

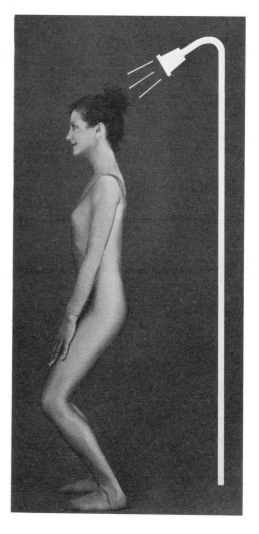

3

Shower Cat Stretch

1. Stand with your feet parallel and shoulder-width apart. Bend your knees and rest your hands on your thighs, back straight and lengthened.

2. Exhale slowly as you contract your abdominal muscles and round your back. Hold the arched position for 3 counts.

Then, with a slow inhalation, resume the straight-back position.

Repetition: Six times

For a massaging effect, point the shower head in the direction of your lower back as you arch and straighten.

(Tip) If you direct the jet to individual parts of your body, switching from hot to cool and back to hot again, it will stimulate your all-over circulation.

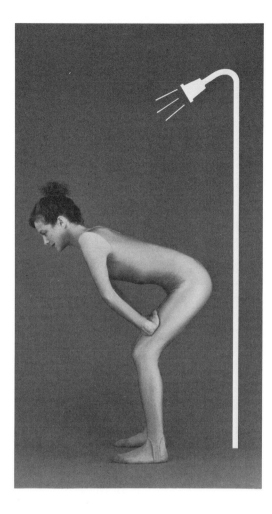

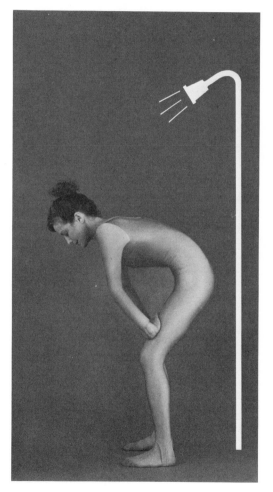

TOWEL TONERS

1

Towel Tilt

1. Stand with your feet comfortably apart. Bend your elbows and hold the towel taut behind your head.

2. Keeping the towel taut and your hips centered, tilt it from side to side.

Repetition: Twelve times to each side

With each towel toner exercise, remember to exhale your breath on the exertion, inhale on the release.

(Tip) Tape makeup hints from magazines inside your mirrored medicine chest or store them with your makeup.

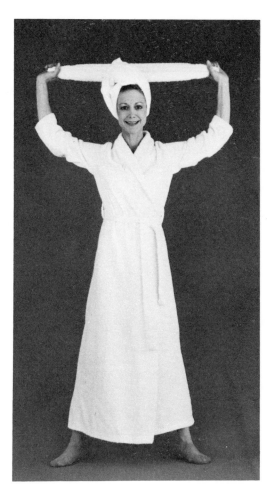

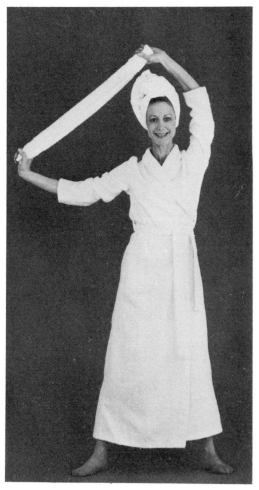

2

Towel Lift

1. Stand with your feet wide apart and parallel. Hold the towel down taut behind your body, arms straight and palms facing forward.

2. Lift and lower your arms, keeping the towel taut. Exhale on each lift.

Repetition: Twenty-four times

(Tip) For painless eyebrow tweezing, stretch the skin taut, then pluck. Less pull, less "ouch."

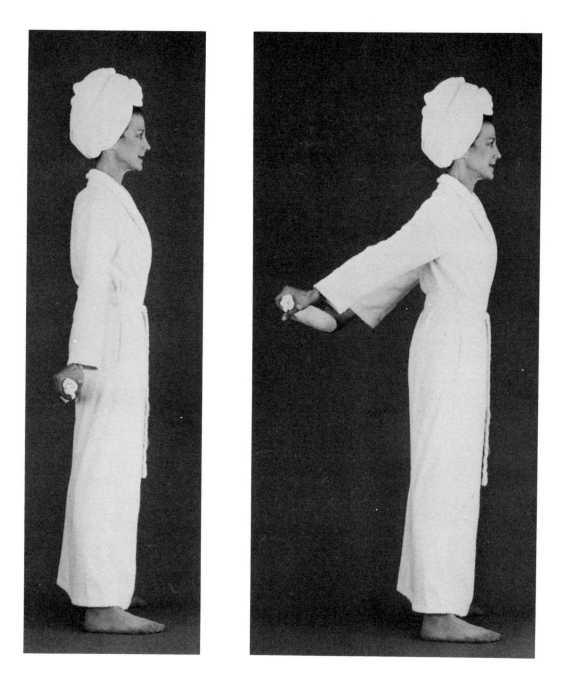

3

Towel Tug

1. Stand with your feet wide apart. Bend your elbows, holding the towel taut behind your neck.

2. Keeping the towel taut, lift your arms until they straighten.

Then bend them to the original position. Exhale on the lift.

Repetition: Twenty-four times

(Tip) Light, heat and air distort a fragrance. If you don't plan to use your perfume or cologne frequently, store it in a cool, dark place. A warm, steamy bathroom will cause it to evaporate more rapidly.

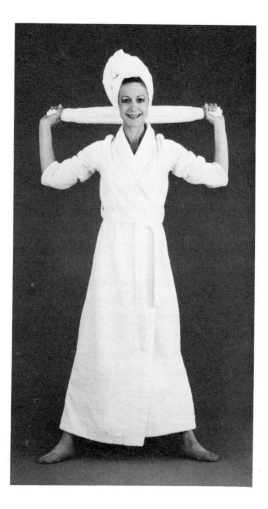

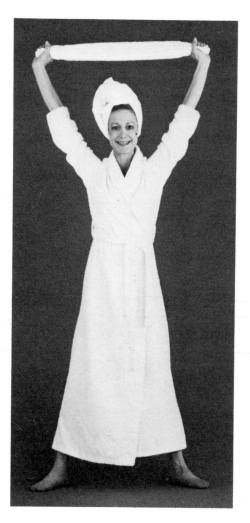

4

SNEAKY EXERCISES

It's possible to "steal" a stretch just about anytime and anywhere. So, too, many exercises can be adapted to slip into your busy day in lieu of your having to adjust your schedule to fit an exercise timetable. Little snippets of exercise . . . an arm curl here, an ankle rotation there are obviously not going to recontour your body or burn countless calories. What these "sneaky" exercises will do is ease tension, stimulate circulation and replace fatigue with renewed energy.

We're all captive to waiting periods and "killing time," be it at the doctor's office, the bank, supermarket or hairdresser. That's where these micromovements come in handy. I even exercise when in the lift. While everyone else is staring at the floor numbers, yours truly is contracting her buttock muscles. The same exercise can be done while riding the bus or Tube to work. In fact, strap-hanging provides the ideal opportunity for bottom-firming. Tighten your buttock muscles and maintain the contraction for several seconds, then release. Repeat again and again, trying to squeeze a bit more forcefully each time. If you don't groan and grimace, I promise, no one will know what you're up to.

Busy working women are nothing less than pros at doing two things simultaneously. They have to be. While on the phone, putting groceries away, or watching television for example, you can punctuate the activity with a stretch or two. It's simply a matter of learning to use everyday situations to best advantage. Try reaching a little higher when looking for something in your kitchen cabinet. Make telephone calls while standing up, so you can twist and turn. Use two full cardboard cartons of salt for weights (they weigh twenty-six ounces) and tone your arms while your pasta cooks. Do knee bends and leg lifts, using your kitchen counter as a ballet barre. Run in place for several minutes while your breakfast coffee is percolating. When driving and stopped for a red light, contract your abdominals and press your spine against the back of the seat. Once you begin conditioning yourself to weave exercise into everyday activities, you'll be surprised how much movement mileage you can get around the clock.

Have you ever contemplated the number of hours you spend talking on the telephone, be it at home or at work? In a lifetime, the figure is truly staggering. Whether you're catching up on frivolous gossip or getting down to serious business, phone time can turn into "tone" time. With just the merest bit of effort, you can exercise more than just your vocal cords. And because of the subtle nature of phone toning, there should be no huffing or puffing to give you away. If, like me, you become a raving maniac when you're put on "hold" for what seems an eternity, phone toners are ideal to assuage irritation. When I'm at my office, involved in an extended conversation, I may slip out of my shoes so that I can flex my feet unencumbered by footwear. But it's hardly necessary. For arm toning, I keep three-pound weights in my desk drawer and use the hand that is not holding the phone for some biceps/triceps exercises. (Just be certain to switch hands in order to give yourself a symmetrical workout.) Naturally, the situation will dictate their practicality. One of my clients, a successful estate agent, emphatically states that knee bends and leg lifts in a cramped Manhattan phone booth simply don't work.

While watching television, in addition to the toners I've suggested, you may also wish to practise some of the exercises I've included in the A.M. and P.M. workouts. The message I'm trying to underscore is that there are truly endless occasions during the course of your day, at home and at work, when you can insert a stretch or two. Take a break to massage your temples, breathe deeply, walk for ten minutes during your lunch hour. Remember, the benefits are cumulative. Fitness is not an overnight goal, it's a lifetime pursuit. By punctuating your day with movement, you make exercise an intrinsic part of your life, adding up to a springier, more vibrant, more comfortable you.

OFFICISES

1

Slouched and Slumped/Sitting Pretty

After long hours of sitting, a chair-bound body tends to slide into a slouch as illustrated. This is particularly apt to occur if your chair lacks proper support. Take pointers from the next photo: Your "sitting bones" in your bottom should be snug in the back of the chair. Stomach, chest, shoulders, neck and head should stack up on top like building blocks. Sit straight and poised. Smile—you're sitting pretty.

(**Tip**) Proteins are a natural and nutritious way to keep your mind performing at its peak level. To keep on a mental roll through the afternoon, make sure you include a protein at lunch, such as 3 to 4 ounces of water-packed tuna, chicken or turkey slices, or a cup of cottage cheese.

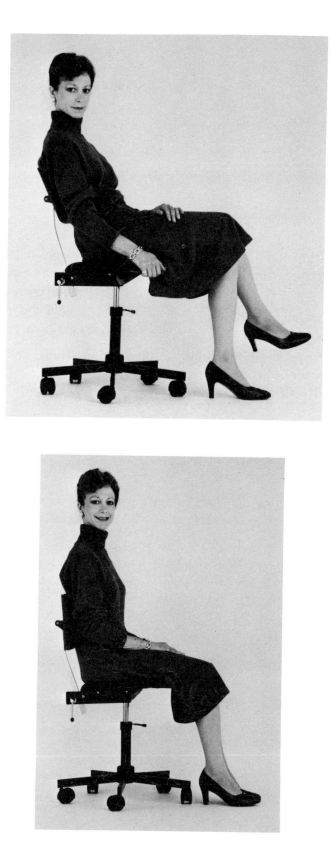

2

Rag Doll

1. Sit upright in your chair, feet parallel and about shoulder-width apart. Relax your arms on your thighs.

2. Inhale deeply, then slowly exhale as you lower your chin and round your back. At the same time, slide your hands down your legs toward your ankles. Release any tension in your neck and shoulders. Hang limply for 6 counts, breathing relaxed. Then slowly inhale and uncurl, vertebra by vertebra, until you resume the original straight-back position.

Repetition: Three times

(**Tip**) Diet lunch bag hint: Instead of bread, wrap cabbage or cos lettuce leaves around a low-calorie sandwich filling (e.g., sliced turkey breast).

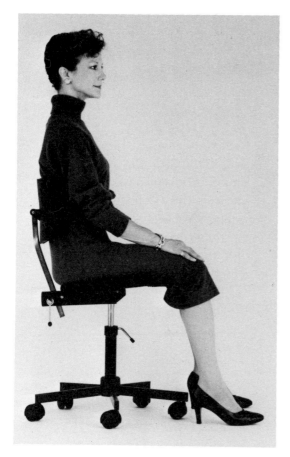

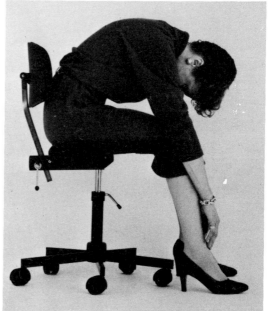

3

Foot Flex

1. Sit tall with your right leg extended in front. Place your hands on the chair for support or relax them at your sides.

2. Keeping the leg lifted, flex and point the foot 8 times. Repeat on the left leg.

Repetition: Two sets on each leg

The harder you flex, the greater stretch you will feel in the calf muscle. This is effective for activating tired legs and feet. To rev up circulation, you can also rotate the foot from the ankle, in a clockwise, then counterclockwise, direction.

(Tip) Feet tend to swell during the day, so it's best to shop for shoes in the afternoon. If shoes need to be "broken in," don't buy them. They'll never really be right.

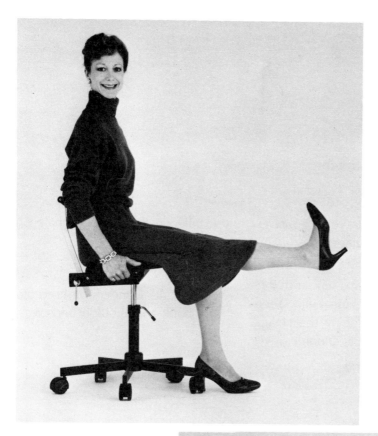

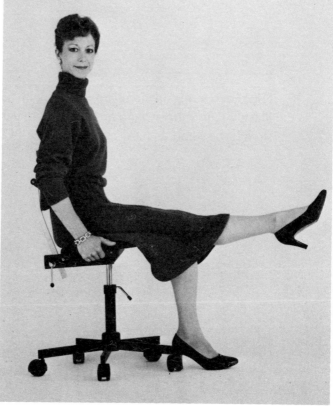

4

Upper Back Stretch

1. Sit tall with your arms extended at shoulder level, palms clasped, facing out.

2. Lift your arms up and then slightly behind your head, keeping the palms facing the ceiling. Lower the arms to shoulder level.

Exhale on the lift and inhale on the release.

Repetition: Ten times

This works wonders on tired upper-back and shoulder muscles.

(Tip) For revving up circulation in the palm and fingers, try the following: Place a tight rubber band around your fingers. Spread fingers apart and stretch the band as hard as you can. Hold five seconds.

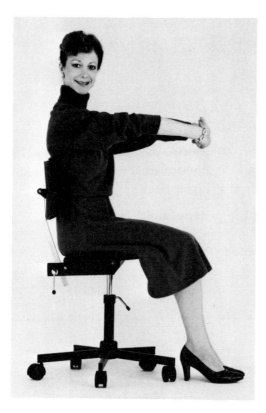

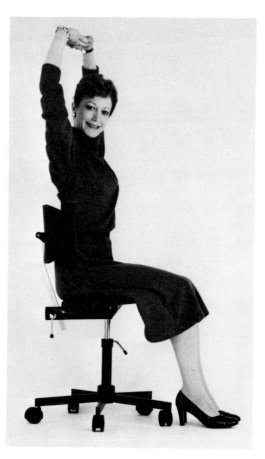

5

Chest Stretch

1. Sit tall with your hands interlaced behind your head, elbows wide open.

2. Inhale as you bring your elbows forward until they are parallel. Then exhale and open them wide to the original position. Feel the stretch across your chest and upper back.

Repetition: Twelve times

(Tip) For a second wind or a quick lift without spoiling your makeup, close your eyes and sprinkle on some mineral water. It adds moisture to your skin and gives you a fresh look.

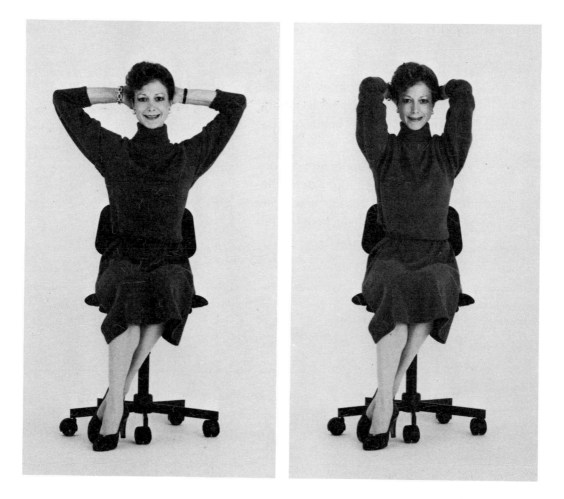

6

Curls

1. Sit with your elbow shoulder height, bent and parallel to the floor. Rest a weight lightly on your shoulder.

2. Keeping the upper arm stationary, exhale as you extend the forearm until it is practically straight. Then inhale, bending it to the starting position.

Repetition: Twenty times on each arm

Whenever you are using weights, make certain that you exhale on the exertion which, in this case, is on the outward extension.

(**Tip**) Making lists is a favourite ploy of busy working women. List-making not only helps with organization but grants a feeling of control.

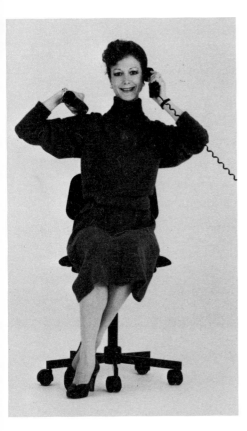

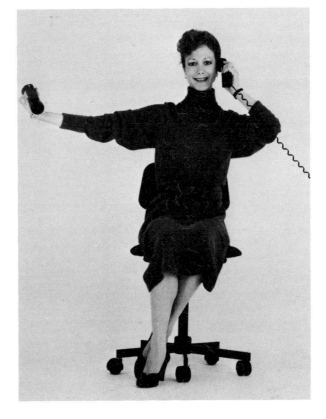

7

Triceps Toner

1. Sit with your elbow bent and pointed upward as much as possible. Hold the weight behind your head, the palm facing forward.

2. Keeping the upper arm stationary, exhale and extend your arm upward, palm forward. Then inhale as you bend the arm to the original position.

Repetition: Twenty times on each arm

(Tip) Try the "rip and read" method. Thumb through publications, tearing out information of special interest. Discard the periodical and keep the articles in a file marked "On the Go Reading." Select several articles to read while commuting to work.

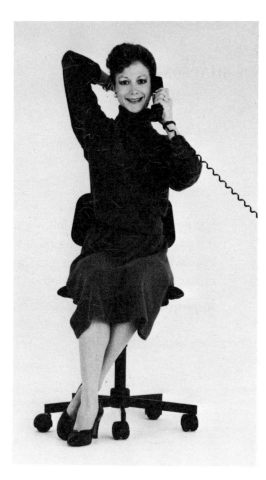

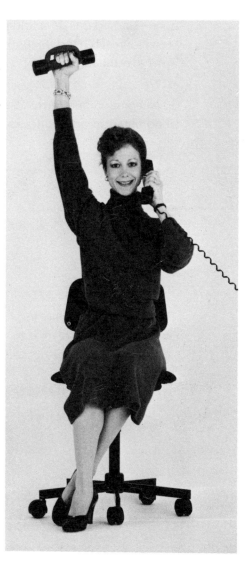

KITCHEN SHAPERS

1

Crossovers

1. Stand with your feet wide apart and parallel. Holding a weight in each hand, extend your arms overhead, crossing at the wrists.

2. Keeping your arms raised, abdominals in and buttocks con-tracted, cross right over left, then left over right. Repeat 16 times. If you wish, you can also do the crossovers behind your body.

Repetition: Two sets

(Tip) If you run or play too hard and don't have an ice pack to soothe the strain, try a bag of frozen vegetables (peas and carrots are ideal) for emergency medicine. It costs less than a chemist's model and moulds well to the body.

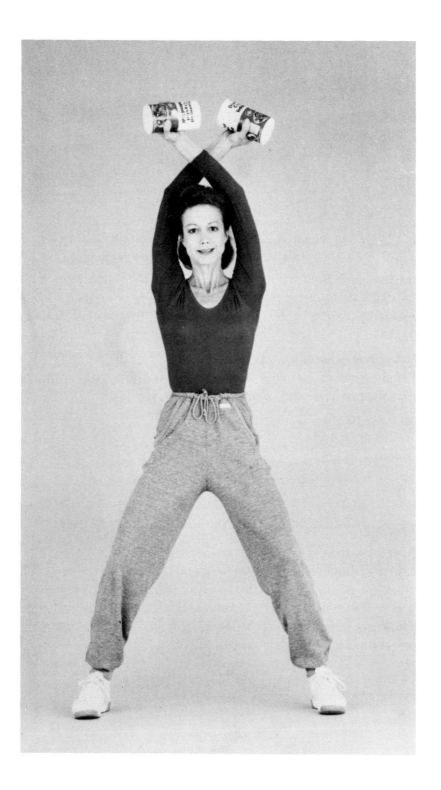

2

Curls

1. Stand with your feet wide apart and parallel. Hold a weight in each hand. Bend your elbows and point them directly forward, resting the weights lightly on each shoulder.

2. Keeping your elbows pointed directly forward and your upper arms stationary, extend your arms forward until they are practically straight. Then bend them to the original position. Repeat 15 times, exhaling with each forward motion. Concentrate on keeping your abdominals tight and your buttocks tucked under.

Repetition: Two complete sets

(Tip) How long can you keep vitamins? High-quality vitamins, handled properly, should have a shelf-life of about three to five years. The bathroom is a poor choice. Better to keep vitamins in the kitchen with dry goods. The refrigerator is a good storage spot for vitamins on hold for future use. Before opening, let containers warm to room temperature to prevent moisture buildup.

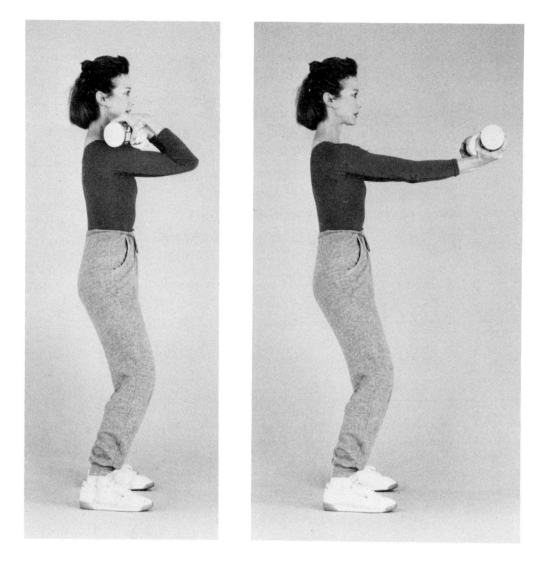

3

Openers

1. Stand with your feet shoulder-width apart and parallel. Extend your arms forward at chest level, a weight in each hand.

2. Open your arms to the sides (avoid locking your elbows). Then close them to the original position. Repeat 12 times, exhaling as you open.

Repetition: Two sets

(**Tip**) Food for good looks. Broccoli is high in vitamin C (for healthy skin, teeth, bones and gums) and A (to grow and maintain skin and hair). It also contains two essential minerals, calcium and iron.

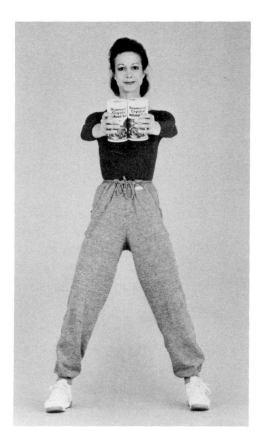

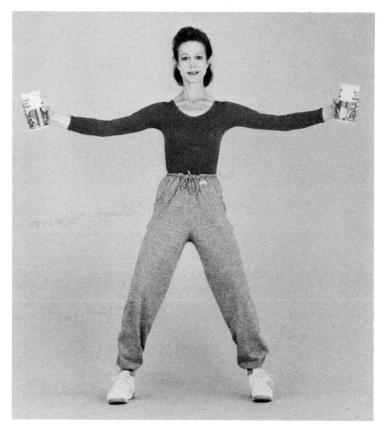

4

Press Backs

1. Stand with your feet comfortably apart and parallel. Hold a weight in each hand, palms facing back.

2. Keeping your arms close to your body, press them back at a moderate tempo. Repeat 20 times, accompanying each backward motion with a short exhalation.

Repetition: Three sets

This one really tightens up the back of the upper arms, one of the first areas to reveal age.

(**Tip**) Three nibbles worth 100 Calories: 5 large prunes, 1 apple, 2 cups of popcorn (no butter).

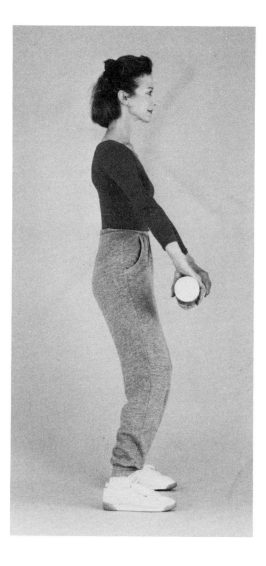
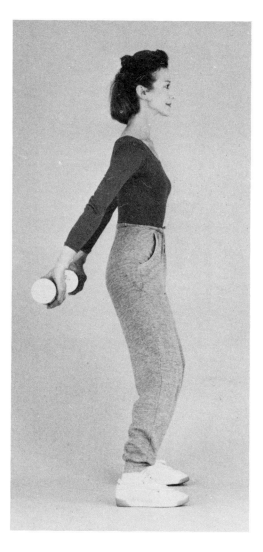

TV TONERS

1

Knee Pulse

1. Sit upright with the soles of your feet together. Rest your hands on your ankles.

2. Maintaining a straight back, press your knees downward 20 times. Keep your breathing natural. Shake out your legs and repeat.

Repetition: Three sets

(Tip) You'll double your accomplishments if you do small tasks while engaged in some other activity.

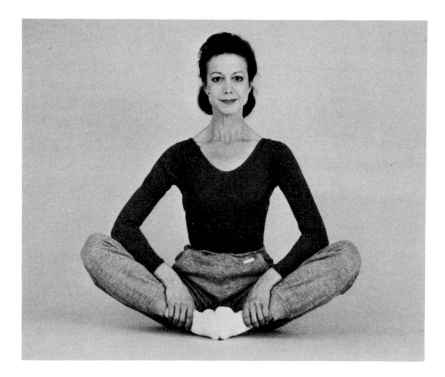

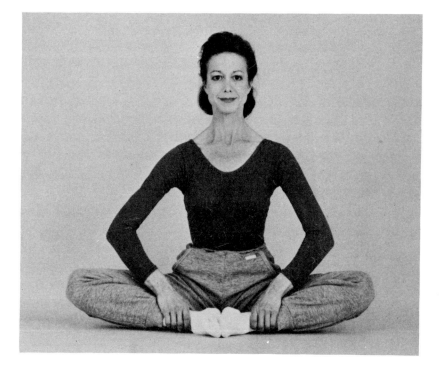

2

Waist Whittler

1. Sit with your feet flat on the floor, knees bent and together. Interlace your hands behind your head, elbows wide open.

2. Exhale and extend your arms up, palms facing the ceiling. Take the time to really feel the stretch in your waist. Then lower your arms to the starting position. Repeat 20 times.

Repetition: Three sets

In order to work your inner thighs as well, squeeze them together each time you straighten your arms.

(Tip) Call to confirm appointments before you leave home or your office to double-check that the dentist, doctor, etc., is running on time.

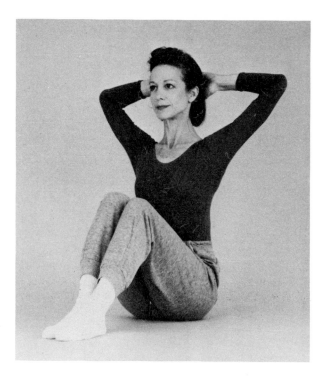

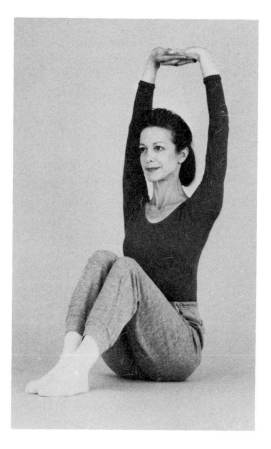

3

Leg Rotations

1. Sit tall with your legs extended to the sides, toes pointed. Rest your hands on your knees.

2. Roll your legs outward as far as you can, then roll them inward, keeping your body lifted and your spine lengthened. Repeat the total movement 10 times. Readjust your legs again so they are as wide apart as possible, then repeat.

Repetition: Three complete sets

In this same position with legs extended and wide apart, you can also flex and point the feet.

(Tip) Anticipate—and prevent—minor and major crises by planning ahead. Stock up on birthday and anniversary cards and appropriate gifts; buy a roll of 100 stamps; hide spare cash in the house for those days when you can't get to the bank.

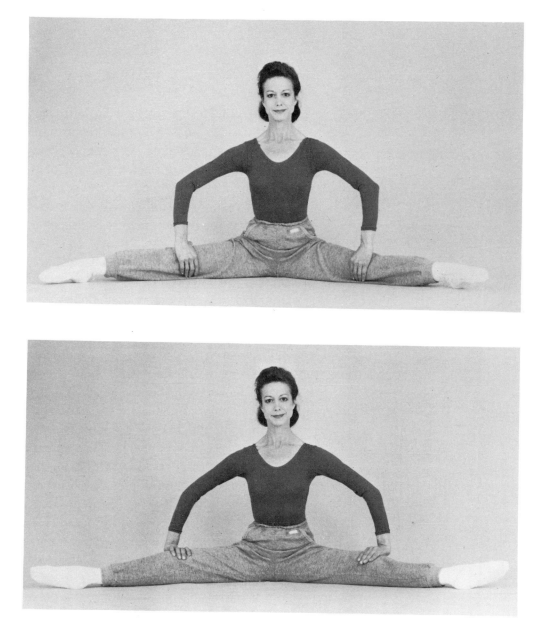

5

P.M.
PICKUP

The P.M. Pickup is designed to zero in on your "disaster areas" while at the same time giving you a quick after-work energy boost. When muscles are neglected, because of inactivity, they shorten and fatty bulges form around them. As the muscles become strong and toned, the bumps and bulges disappear, or at least become less obvious. Toned-up muscles take up less room than flaccid, lazy ones. Providing you're consistent, results from this time-efficient, body-defining-refining routine will appear in approximately four weeks, leaving you sleeker and more flexible as well.

If you're satisfied with your present shape (lucky you), this routine of fast flab fixes can help you maintain your attractive proportions. Should you be among the satisfied few, remember gravity is busy at work each minute of every day. Your buttocks, abdominals, upper arms, etc. are all susceptible to its ruthless tugging. It's up to you to fight that constant pull downward. One way to challenge gravity is to keep your body strong and toned. By so doing, you can look far younger than your actual years.

What exactly are your figure trouble spots? There's no better way to answer that question than to take a thorough look at yourself in a full length mirror . . . naked, of course. Whatever the flaw or flaws may be, there's no need to accept them as your permanent figure fate. Most problems can be considerably improved. While dieting can and does change your appearance by reducing those extra pounds, only exercise can "cure" your figure liabilities by remoulding your shape to its correct and most attractive proportions. Think of exercise as the precision tool that will sculpt your body and speed up sleekness.

For this segment, I've selected some of my favourite figure-contouring exercises. And because I'm well aware that working women do not have endless hours to devote to body-sculpting endeavours, I've chosen exercises that deliver maximum results in minimum time. Before you begin, be sure to warm up. You might want to jump rope or run in place for several minutes in order to activate your blood flow. If so, be certain that you use appropriate footwear and that the surface on which you work is properly cushioned.

The P.M. Pickup can be used in many ways. Practice it several days a week (five, for best results) for overall contouring, or, you can select only those exercises that particularly address your trouble spots. As for the recommended repetitions, if you wish to pour on more steam, by all means do so, providing you increase the numbers gradually. Or, you can further challenge yourself by adding ankle weights. In addition, when time allows, you can extend this ten-minute routine by combining it with the A.M. Awakener.

When I exercise, music is a must. Even running is more pleasurable with my trusty Walkman. Music helps me move with greater ease and adds considerable enjoyment to my workout time. I use a variety of music . . . rock, jazz, classical, or even the scores from favourite Broadway shows. It depends on my mood. You might prefer the Beatles one day and Beethoven the next. Choose whatever appeals to you—that's what matters most. Also, try to exercise in front of a full-length mirror. By observing your alignment as you move, you will maximize the effectiveness of your workout time.

Many women claim they're simply too exhausted and "wiped out" after work to exercise. Indeed, time restraints can make regular evening workouts impossible to manage. For others, however, a short P.M. routine can serve as the ideal antidote to after-work exhaustion. It can enable you to tackle the evening's activities with restored strength and enthusiasm. In fact, when you're at your most fatigued from job-related frustrations, a few minutes of after-work exercise can give your body and spirit a greater lift than a glass of champagne.

PM PICKUP

1

Arms and Bosom

1. Sit upright with your ankles crossed. Hold a weight (2–5 pounds) behind your head, elbows wide apart.

2. Exhale as you extend your arms upward until they are practi-

cally straight. Bend them to resume the starting position.

Repetition: Twenty-four times

(Tip) Jogging, running or doing aerobics without a bra can cause the ligaments in the breast to weaken and sag. A sports bra should have no seams across the nipple and should minimize your profile in order to protect against tissue-tearing bounce.

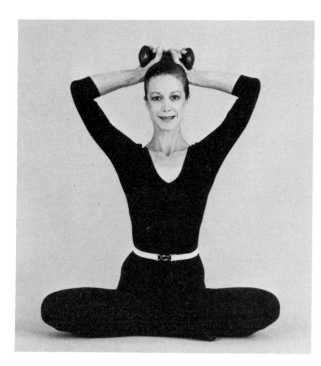

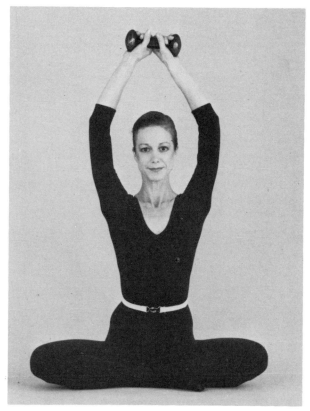

2

Waist

1. Sit upright with your legs extended to the sides, feet pointed and turned out. Interlace your hands behind your head, elbows wide apart.

2. Bend directly sideways from your waist to the right, trying to tilt as far as possible without lifting your left buttock off the floor. Return to centre, lifing high through your upper torso in order to lengthen your spine and feel the stretch in your waist. Repeat to the left side. Repeat 10 times to each side, exhaling as you stretch, inhaling as you lift.

Repetition: Two complete sets

Don't let your elbows come together; try to keep them wide apart throughout the exercise.

(Tip) To minimize a thicker waistline, don't wear colours that divide at the waist—for example, a pink blouse with a black skirt.

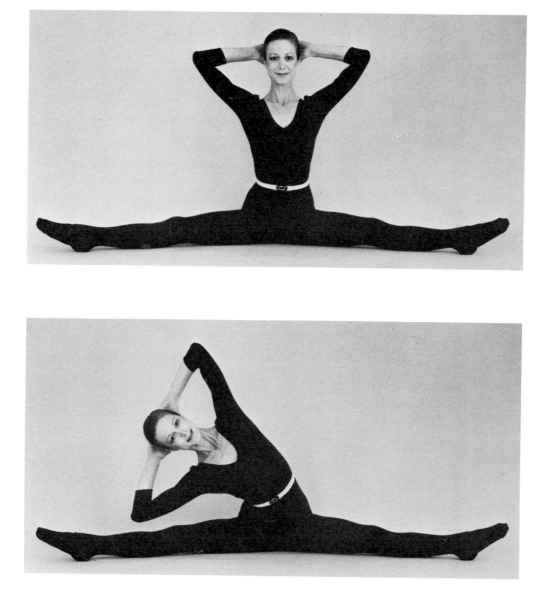

3

Abdominal Muscles

1. Lie on your back with the soles of your feet together and close to your body. Interlace your hands behind your neck, elbows pointed toward the ceiling.

2. Contract your abdominal muscles and press the small of your back into the floor as you lift until your shoulders clear the floor, elbows pointed forward. Lower a bit, then lift again, exhaling with each forward pulse. Repeat the upward pulsing motion 12 times. Then roll completely back to the floor.

Repetition: Four sets

If you find your abdomen begin to push out before you have completed a set, roll back to the floor and contract again. It is preferable to do fewer repeats correctly (with abdominal control) than more, poorly positioned. If you wish to relax between sets, hug your knees to your chest.

(Tip) With any abdomen-toning exercise, the moment the small of your back leaves the floor, your abdominal muscles have passed the buck to your hip flexors.

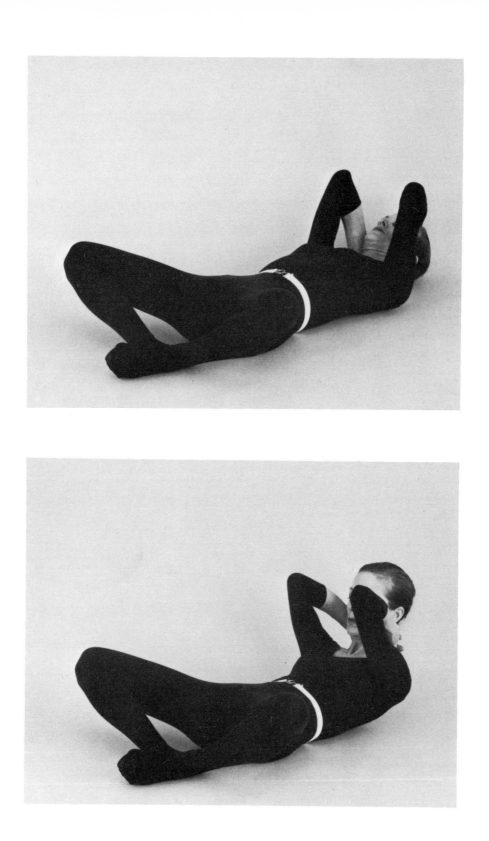

4

Inner Thighs

1. Lie on your right side, rest on your right elbow. Extend your right leg to the side in line with your upper body. Flex the foot and turn the heel up. Bend your left leg, resting your left foot on the floor behind your right thigh and place your hand on your knee.

2. Keeping your heel turned up, lift and lower (not quite to the floor) your leg. Repeat 24 times on each side.

Repetition: Three complete sets

Use ankle weights only if you are able to execute the exercise with proper alignment and control. When you are using weights, the exhalation should always accompany the exertion.

(**Tip**) Go for a professional leg waxing before attempting it on your own. You'll familiarize yourself with the procedure and get a feel for the proper wax temperature.

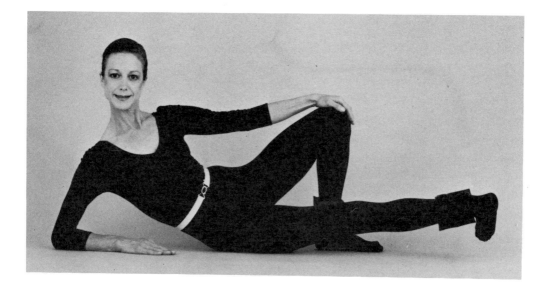

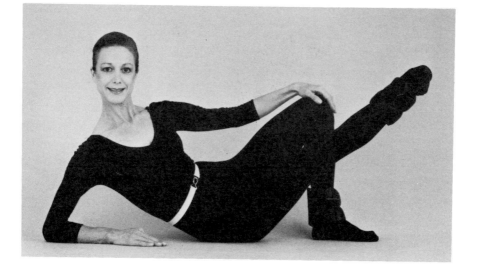

5

Outer Thigh

1. Lie on your right side. Use your right elbow and left hand to support your torso. Bend your right knee. Extend your left leg to the side at hip level and in line with your body. Make certain the knee is facing forward and the foot is flexed as much as possible.

2. Lift your leg as high as you can without changing the position of the knee and foot. Lower it again to hip level. Repeat 24 times on each side.

Repetition: Three complete sets

(Tip) How you apply a moisturizer to your legs can be as important as what's in it. Always rub moisturizer downward on the legs, toward the feet, not against the direction of hair growth. Rubbing creams and lotions up into the small, porelike follicles can cause inflammation.

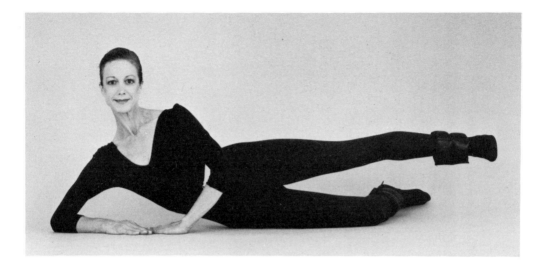

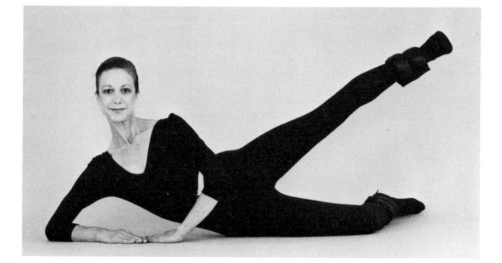

6

Hips

1. Lie on your back with your right leg extended in front. Rest your left foot on your right knee, facing the knee to the ceiling. Place your hands on your waist.

2. Keeping your shoulders stationary and the foot in place, lower your knee as far to the right, then as far to the left as you can. Repeat the total movement 12 times on each leg keeping your breathing normal and relaxed.

Repetition: Two complete sets

(**Tip**) Large hips are generally genetically influenced. To camouflage them, use above-the-waist details. Wear skirts that are long enough to balance your hips—a skirt that's too short emphasizes your width.

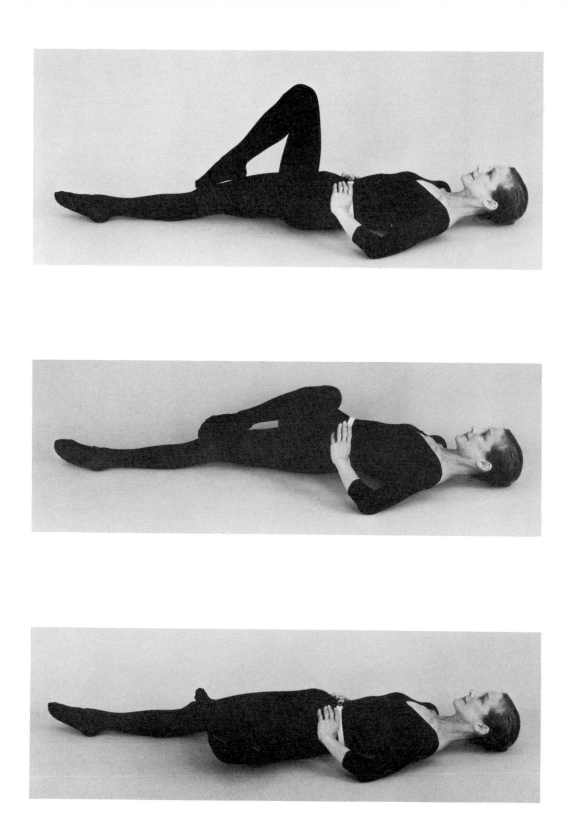

7

Buttocks

1. Lie on your right side with your right knee bent. Place your left hand on the floor for support and your right hand against your head. Extend your left leg to the side in line with your body. Flex the foot and rest only your toes on the floor. Point the heel up and the knee down.

2. Exhale and lift your leg as high as possible without changing the position of the knee and heel. Then inhale as you lower it, touching the foot to the floor. Repeat 24 times on each leg.

Repetition: Three complete sets

(Tip) Stair-climbing (try two steps at a time) can help to lift drooping buttocks.

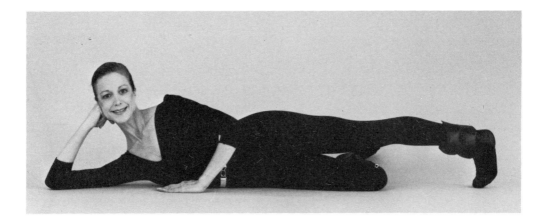

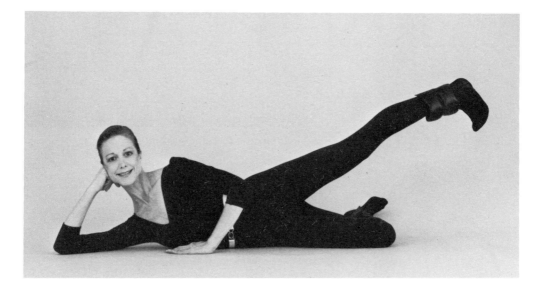

6

RELAXERCISES

Unwinding is as essential to a working woman's well-being as exercise. Because your days are jam-packed and often pressured, the need to restore your energy must never be overlooked or underestimated. The stress and demands from multiple responsibilities and roles—mother, friend, careerist, wife—can affect the quality of your work, your ability to relax and your appetite to enjoy life. It can take its toll on your looks, your body and your emotions. Stress can truly "sneak" up on you.

Relaxation . . . You need it . . . You deserve it . . . Make it a regular part of your day. Relaxation is very different from sleep. It's beneficial daily to give renewed vigour to activities, and also to adjust your attitude toward frustrations and irritations. Learning to relax can increase your self-control, enabling you to reassess your problems and approach them more positively.

We're all subject to tension, that involuntary tightening of muscles and nerves that can make us feel tired and cranky (and look it as well). But how can we best cope with stress and the endless demands placed upon us? The bottom line is reserving time every day to do something relaxing. Stretching is one of the most important—and easiest—things you can do. Slow, controlled, gentle movements can ease the overworked, the keyed-up, even the insomniac.

Now, I'm not claiming these Relaxercises are going to magically dissolve all your problems. What I do know is that in only a few minutes' time, they loosen and relax tense muscles and tendons to such a degree that you immediately feel better and more equipped to deal with your problems. By incorporating them into your personal exercise plan, you will learn to identify just where tension grabs and how you feel when it's gone. And because of their anxiety-reducing affect, they will energize you as well. Also, if you have difficulty falling asleep, these Relaxercises can help your body slow down, thus making you more receptive to sweet dreams.

No matter what your job may be, there's no escaping stress. What's important is dealing with it—defusing it. Stress need not always be negative. It can work for you in a positive way by stimulating action and the energy to attack everyday challenges. Stress only becomes negative, and therefore harmful, when these challenges provoke discouragement, anxiety and a sense of being out of control and unable to cope. This puts one in a state of *distress,* which is truly harmful and can result in insomnia, exhaustion and in severe cases burnout that can lead to breakdown. The problem is knowing the line between stress that is beneficial, that allows you to work to your fullest, and stress overload that is detrimental to your health. One key to working and living at your peak is recognizing your personal stress tolerance, and the point at which arousal ceases to be positive.

No two women react to stress in quite the same way. Some develop mild physical symptoms. In others, subtle mood changes appear as common early warning signals. A woman may find that she has less patience with people or with problems that she usually deals with quite easily. Or she may make mistakes in relatively straightforward tasks. Tension also can interfere with decision-making, problem-solving or the ability to express oneself with ease and clarity.

I frequently witness in my clients varying physical manifestations that are stress-provoked. Some women experience pain in the lower back, others across the shoulders. Many complain of gastrointestinal upset or headaches from mild to migraine. That's why it's so important to become aware of what affects *you* personally and to recognize your own anxieties and reactions to stressful situations. This will allow you to deal with stress positively in lieu of having it clobber you. So too, reducing stress also depends on finding a technique that appeals to your personality and lifestyle. An action-oriented person, for example, might have a difficult time relaxing if forced to sit still for twenty minutes repeating a mantra, while a series of slow yoga postures might work ideally.

When practising the Relaxercises as a complete routine, slip into something that allows for ease of movement—underwear, sweats or nothing at all. Try, if possible, to retreat to a spot where you won't be disturbed. Above all, take your time, giving special attention to proper breathing technique. Inhale deeply through your nose, and exhale through your mouth. Never rush the process or force the movements. There should be no pain or strain. Work toward achieving a sense of your entire body giving way to gravity as if melting into nothingness. Establish a calm and serene image in your mind, one that will allow you to just "let go."

As I noted earlier in the book, I find the relaxation exercises particularly effective as a follow-up to a soothing evening bath. For me, combining the two almost always serves as my insurance policy for a good night's sleep. On the other hand, the exercises need not be practised as a complete segment. One of my clients, an illustrator, finds the deep-breathing exercise particularly helpful while she awaits her much dreaded dental checkup. Remember, it need not be practiced while lying on the floor as illustrated; it can be done in a chair as well. One client claims it lessens her trepidation during airplane takeoffs and landings. Another client, a marketing research whiz, finds "The Dangle" effective as a detenser before she delivers an important presentation.

Working women experience the same career stresses that men do, but few are willing to relinquish any of their traditional roles. We've just added new stresses to old ones. Much to our detriment, we tend to make everything a number-one priority and thus we find we're always too exhausted to take time out to relax. But you can, and you must, pull your tension plugs when you feel you're overloading your system. Through regular practice of the brief relaxation segment that follows, you will be better equipped to combat the effects of stress on your mind and body.

RELAXERCISES

1

The Dangle

1. Stand with your feet wide apart and slightly turned out. Relax your arms at your sides.

2. Take 4 slow counts to round your back while exhaling your breath. Allow your knees to bend and your arms to hang limply. Let your head become a weight at the end of your spine. Hold this limp position for 10 counts keeping your breathing relaxed. Then inhale slowly and using your abdominal muscles, roll up one vertebra at a time. Keep your chin to your chest until you have uncurled completely.

Repetition: Two times

For this exercise as well as all the Relaxercises, inhale through the nose and exhale through the mouth.

(Tip) The best eating strategy during periods of stress is frequent small meals. Long periods when your stomach is empty allows acid to do the most damage.

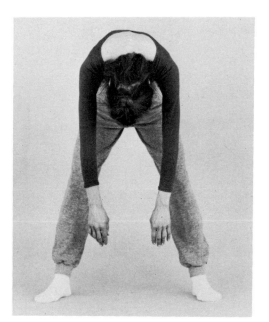

2

Spine Dekinker

1. Sit with your ankles crossed. Place your hands on the floor, elbows bent to the sides. Lower your head and round your back.

2. Keeping your back rounded, press gently downward as you exhale. Then press away from the floor lifting several inches as you inhale. Repeat the total down-up motion 8 times. Roll up, starting at the base of your spine until you have uncurled completely.

Repetition: Three sets

(Tip) To relieve tension behind your eyelids, press gently under the brow bone with your thumbs. Then lightly massage the sides of your nose next to your eyes.

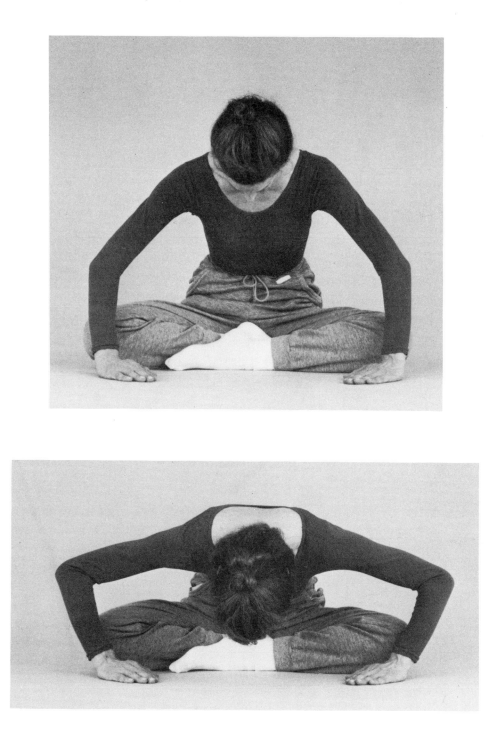

3

Upper Body Stretch

1. Sit on your heels with your knees together. Interlace your hands behind your body.

2. Take 4 slow counts to lower your body as you simultaneously lift your arms behind. Keep your chin tucked into your chest. Hold for 4 counts, breathing normally.

Then, inhale and take 4 counts to lower your arms and lift your body to the original position. Try to time the exhalation to the rounding of the back and the inhalation to the lift.

Repetition: Four times

(Tip) Yoga is a movement technique that is very compatible with mental relaxation. For yoga to be effective, you must be willing to surrender to the rhythm of your body movements.

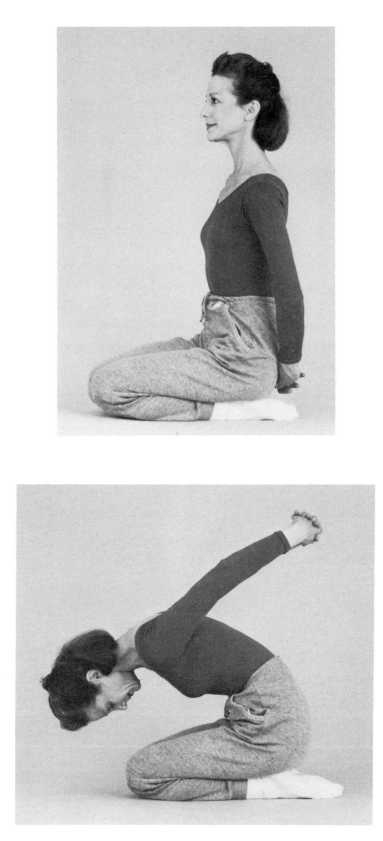

4

Spine Lengthener

1. Sit tall with your ankles crossed, hands relaxed on your knees.

2. Lower your head and round your back, placing your forearms on the floor in front of your knees. Stretch forward, lengthening your spine, as you slide your hands forward. Keep your elbows slightly bent and your chin low. Hold the stretch for 6 counts breathing slowly and deeply. Uncurl, vertebra by vertebra, until you resume the original upright position.

Repetition: Four times

(Tip) For a relaxation break, elevate your feet and cover your eyes with cool, wet tea bags; chamomile is especially soothing.

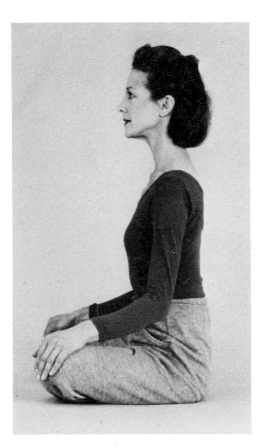

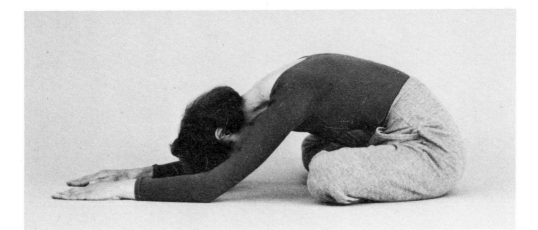

5

Double Leg Rock

1. Lie on your back with your legs extended up. Interlace your hands behind your slightly bent knees.

2. Gently ease your legs toward your chest. Repeat the forward rocking motion 8 times. Exhale as you draw the knees toward you; inhale as they release slightly. Lower your legs and hug your knees to your chest for a count of 6.

Repetition: Three sets

(Tip) The relaxing effects of carbohydrates are even greater later in the evening when you naturally begin to tire. A small carbohydrate snack thirty minutes before you want to sleep may help nudge you along.

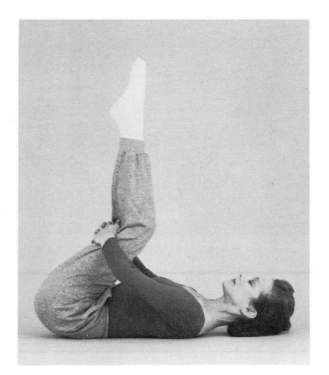

6

Knee Hug

1. Lie on your back with your ankles crossed, knees wide apart. Rest your hands on your ankles.

2. Draw your knees toward your body by gently pulling on your ankles. Maintain the "hug" for 8 counts, breathing slowly and deeply. Release by letting your elbows straighten slightly.

Repetition: Six times

(Tip) The trancelike state induced by hypnosis or meditation does not resemble sleep but is a separate physiological state of enhanced relaxation. Both techniques can be effective in relieving stress if taught by a medically qualified instructor.

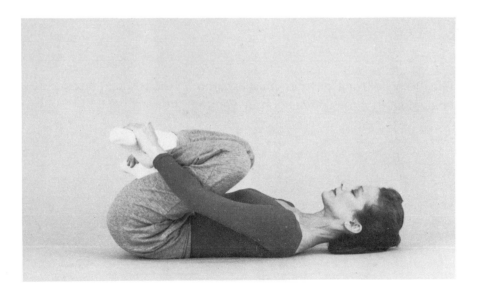

7

Deep Breathing

1. Lie on your back, legs extended in front. Rest your hands on your rib cage. Close your eyes (if you wish) and try to release any muscle tension.

2. Inhale deeply through your nose, taking 4 counts to "inflate." Let your breath flow upward into your chest area as you feel an expansion of your upper torso. Next, take 4 counts to exhale, contracting your abdominal muscles until the air is spent. With the abdominal contraction you should feel the lower part of your back making solid contact with the floor.

Repetition: One minute minimum

Try to maintain a continuous rhythm. There should be no tension, except in the abdomen, when breathing out. In addition to relaxing you, this exercise will enable you to control your breath and increase your lung capacity.

(Tip) To be relaxing, exercise must be approached as something done for enjoyment, not for competition or constant improvement.

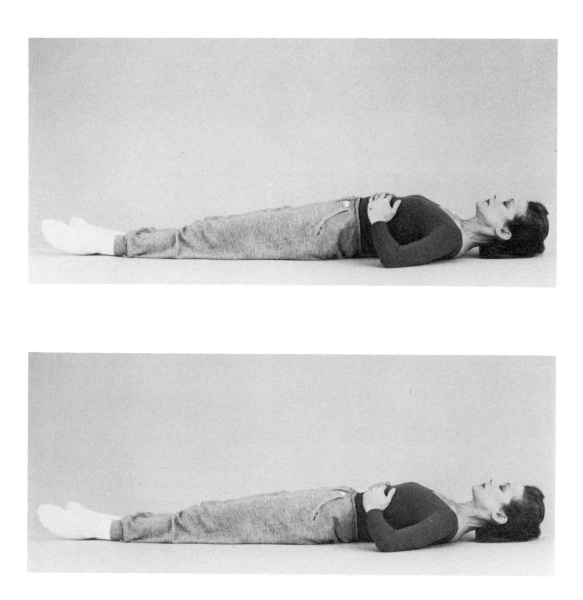

8

Temple Massage

1. Sit with your ankles crossed or lie on your back with your eyes closed. Place your middle three fingers on your temples.

2. Very slowly, circle your fingers outward 10 times, then reverse direction and circle them inward. Keep your breathing relaxed and deep.

Repetition: Two complete sets

(Tip) A facial steam is a relaxing and easy at-home skin beautifier. Fill a basin with hot tap water, tenting a towel over your head and it. Hold your face over the warm mist for five minutes, making certain not to lean too close.

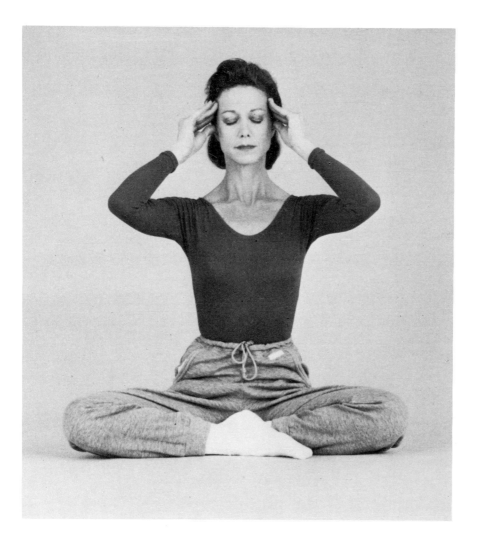

SECTION

II

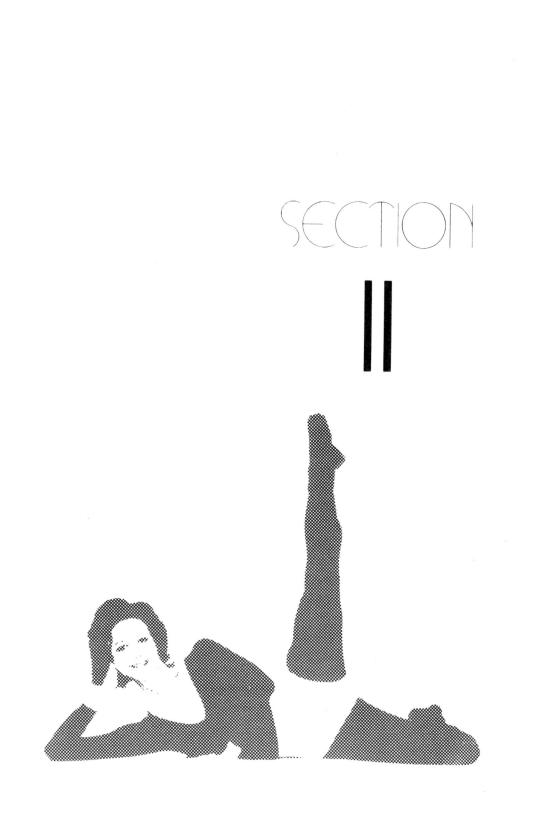

The condition known as "secretary spread" respects no corporate hierarchy or job description. The sedentary set—therapists, editors, receptionists, etc. all share a common concern for one figure spot in particular—the buttocks. Ideally, your buttocks should be smooth, curved and firm. But if your job has you seat-bound, a droopy derriere is probably your major figure liability.

Because of the difficulty of bringing this area back to an attractive, healthful condition once it has begun to deteriorate, the best advice is to concentrate your efforts on keeping your buttocks firm and strong through regular conditioning exercises. The health and shape of the buttocks are governed by a fundamental principle enunciated by Hippocrates, referred to as the father of medicine: "That which is used develops, that which is not used wastes away."

My suggestion would be to keep off your buttocks, but that's hardly a realistic recommendation. The sedentary working woman must try, however, to incorporate as much movement into her day as possible. Devise every conceivable excuse to get out of your chair. Take the phone call standing up. Walk at lunchtime. Or, if you can, deliver your interoffice memos by hand. *Stand,* whenever the occasion allows. The reason for this is that sitting for too long

7

PRESCRIPTION FOR WOMEN WHO ARE SEAT-BOUND

compresses the buttock tissues and cuts down on vital circulation. This causes the buttocks (and hips) to widen and spread out of proportion.

Should you have no choice but to sit, it's important to prevent your buttocks from spreading unnecessarily. Most women tend to sit with their bodies improperly placed. Instead of sitting up and slightly forward, they slouch and lean back on the largest part of their buttocks. Try instead, to sit on your "sitting bones." What exactly are these bones and where are they? They are two small, curved bones that extend down from the lower edge of the pelvis and underlie the pads of muscle and fat in the buttocks. You can feel them by pressing your fingers into the bottom of each buttock. You must learn to sit on them to keep your pelvis properly erect. By so doing, you will also strengthen your lower back. And by all means, refrain from crossing your legs at the thighs.

Contracted voluntarily throughout the day, whenever and wherever possible, your "rear view" will benefit noticeably. Keep in mind, as well, if you're sitting for most of the day, the chair you sit on should support you correctly. Try to select a chair appropriate to your body proportions. Your chair should buttress your lower back and hold your body upright. When seated with your knees bent, calves and thighs forming right angles, your feet should rest firmly on the floor. Proper seat depth should allow your back to reach the back of the chair. For a chair that is too deep, try using a pillow to shorten the depth. Finally, bear in mind that sitting properly does not mean you must sit in a rigid, at-attention posture. On the contrary, you should be relaxed and comfortable.

I encourage women with sedentary occupations to walk as much as possible. There's no such thing as an "ideal" exercise, but walking comes close. It can qualify as an aerobic activity and best of all, it can be woven into most women's daily routine. For walking to be aerobic, you must walk with authority. Step out, swing your arms, hold your head up high and breathe deeply. Generally, I recommend a minimum of twenty minutes, at least three days a week. As you progress with your walking programme, your stamina will naturally increase. My clients who include walking in their regular fitness plan relate that their fatigue and stress are considerably reduced. This in turn results in increased energy and productivity. One of my clients, a scriptwriter, makes it a practice to get out of her taxi ten blocks away from her office in order to incorporate some exercise in what might otherwise be a glued-to-her-chair day. Walking to work is a favourite solution for many of my Manhattan clients, who find they are simply unable to schedule at-home workouts on a regular basis.

They walk in plimsolls and change to more appropriate footwear once they arrive at their destination.

Unable to walk to work? You might consider forfeiting your seat on the bus or subway in order to stand. Just balancing, by contracting your buttock muscles, is an exercise in itself. Or, if you drive to work, when you stop for a red light, tighten your buttock muscles and hold until the light (not you) turns green. Keep in mind that bucket seats look better than they feel. They curl your back and shoulders forward causing strain on your muscles. It's a good idea to fill in the hollow with a back rest that keeps your back flat. So too, be sure the seat is close enough to the steering wheel so you don't have to stretch in order to reach it.

A few words about cellulite, that orange-peel skin often found on women's buttocks. (Some women get heavy concentration on the thighs and the backs of the upper arms.) Call it cellulite or anything else, according to most physicians it's basically just plain old fat. So if it's just fat, why does cellulite look so bumpy and unattractive? Certain cells in the body have the capacity to store enormous amounts of fat and about half of the body's fat is deposited in these cells immediately beneath the skin. Strands of fibrous tissue connect the skin to deeper tissue layers and also separate the fat-cell compartments. When the fat cells increase in size, this apparently causes the compartments of fat to bulge and produce a waffled appearance of the skin.

Experts seem to concur that if you store fat, you're more likely to develop this kind of tissue than if you stay lean. In order to improve this condition, it will take dedication and commitment to burning it off. If you have cellulite, you probably need to reduce your body's fat reserve. Dieting coupled with exercise is the recommended line of attack. Dancing, running, cycling, swimming are all good exercises for burning off fat, but the best, according to many physicians, is walking. The reason being that when you walk, the buttock and thigh muscles are used in a pulling motion that greatly helps firm up the areas most prone to cellulite. Naturally, the intensity of the muscle contractions and their benefit depend on the speed with which you walk and for how long.

The exercises included in this section are expressly designed to firm, tone and strengthen the buttocks, while promoting better circulation of blood to the area. And because of the nature of the movements I have selected for this segment, the hips and thighs will benefit as well. The entire routine should take approximately ten minutes to complete. Try to practice it regularly, five days a week, for best results. Be sure when practicing these seven exercises, as well as any other "derriere defining" movements in this book, that you place extra emphasis on contracting the buttock muscles tightly. Take the time to really "squeeze."

You might want to extend this regimen by choosing from some of the hip- and buttock-firming movements included in other sections as well. In addition, you may decide to supplement this segment with exercises from Chapter 9, which concentrates on correcting postural problems that result from prolonged sitting. You can do both routines from start to finish or select only those exercises you care to concentrate on. By combining both, you will be able to mix and match the exercises to form a variety of effective buttock-toning routines.

Here's looking at you . . . BOTTOMS UP!

1

Buttock Squeeze

1. Lie on your stomach with your legs extended and together. Bend your elbows and rest your right hand on top of your left. Rest your chin on top of your hand.

2. Contract your buttock muscles tightly and maintain the contraction for 5 counts, then release.

Repetition: Eight times

This "squeeze" can be done while sitting or standing as well.

(Tip) To enhance a walking workout, add hand weights—beginning with one pound and working up slowly. Ankle weights for walking are not recommended.

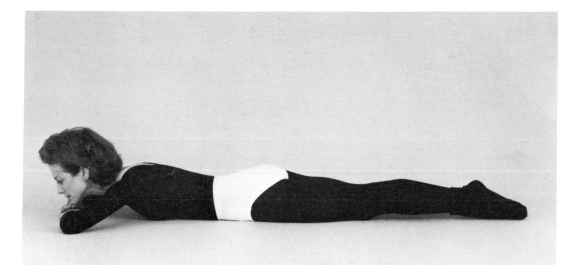

2

Buttock Lift

1. Lie on your back with your knees bent. Place your feet on the floor, slightly more than hip-width apart and parallel. Place your hands behind your head, elbows wide open.

2. Contract your abdominal muscles into a "tuck" position. Tilt your pelvis upward as you tighten and lift your buttocks several inches off of the floor. Do not raise your waist. In this lifted position, contract your buttock muscles, pressing upward slightly, then release the intensity as you lower just a bit. Repeat the squeeze-release bit. Repeat the squeeze-release 20 times, keeping the motion small and controlled. Then roll down, releasing your lower back and buttocks to the floor.

Repetition: Four sets

Exhale with each upward movement and concentrate on keeping your abdomen pulled in. You can hug your knees to your chest between sets to release any muscle fatigue.

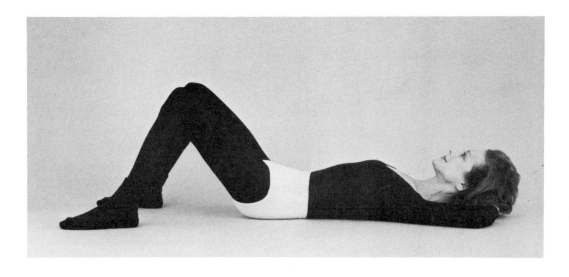

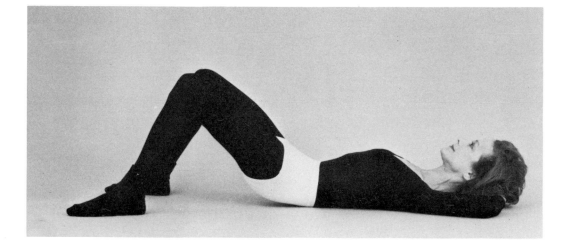

3

Knee Rolls

1. Lie on the floor with your knees bent over your waist. Rest your arms on the floor slightly away from your body, or you may extend them at shoulder level.

2. Keeping your knees together throughout, lower them to the left, trying to touch your left knee to the floor. Your right shoulder should remain in place. Return centre and extend your legs up as you contract your abdominal muscles and exhale your breath. Bend your knees and lower them to the right. The motion is: roll-centre-extend-bend. Remember to inhale on the roll and exhale on the leg extension.

Repetition: Twelve times to each side

(**Tip**) The "bottom line" for buttock rehabilitation is squeeze tight whenever you can.

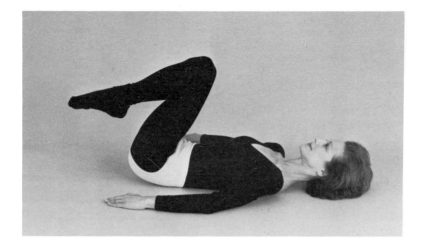

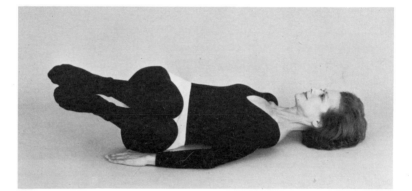

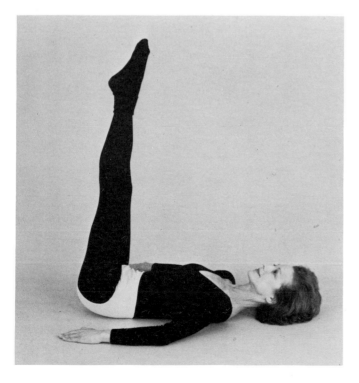

125

4

Knee Tap

1. Lie on your right side and prop your head against your right hand. Bend your right leg, aligning your thigh with your upper body. Rest your left knee on the floor, foot raised. Use your left hand for additional support.

2. Extend your leg up and forward, keeping the toes pointed and the knee facing down. Tap the knee back to the floor before you extend the leg to the side at shoulder level. Repeat the for-ward-tap-side-tap sequence 10 times on each leg.

Repetition: Three sets on each side

With each leg extension, make certain that you exhale your breath and tighten your buttock muscles. Try to keep the rest of your body still and your abdominal muscles contracted.

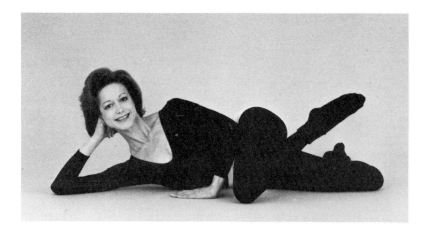

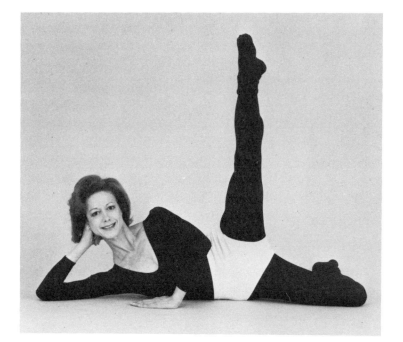

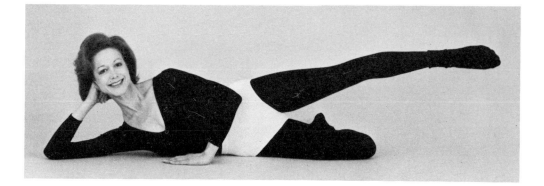

5

Diagonal Lift

1. Lie on your back with your left leg extended in front. Bend your right knee and place the foot on the floor, tilting the knee slightly to the right. Rest your hands on your waist.

2. Lift your left leg diagonally to the right, toes pointed. Then lower it. Repeat 20 times exhaling with each lift. Repeat with the right leg.

Repetition: Two sets on each leg

Try to isolate the leg by keeping the rest of your body as stationary as possible.

(Tip) Strong gluteus maximus muscles prevent excessive lumbar spinal curve (swayback) and reduce fatigue when you stand for long periods of time.

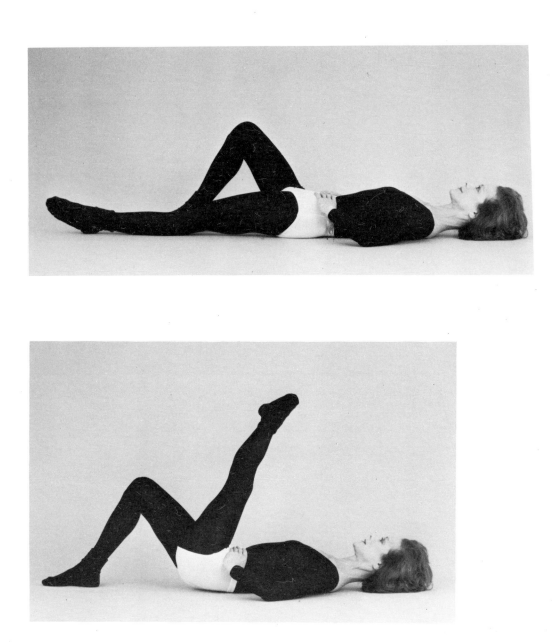

6

Bottom Firmer

1. Lie on your stomach with your legs extended. Bend your elbows and rest your right hand on top of your left. Rest your chin on top of your hand. Without raising your hipbone from the floor, lift your left leg, toes pointed.

2. Keeping the leg raised and the hipbone in contact with the floor, bend and straighten the leg 12 times. Lower the leg and repeat on the right. Exhale on the stretch, inhale on the bend.

Repetition: Three complete sets

This exercise is only effective if you tightly contract your buttock muscles each time the leg straightens. Should you feel any strain in your lower back, check to make certain your hipbone is in place. If back discomfort persists, do not continue with this exercise.

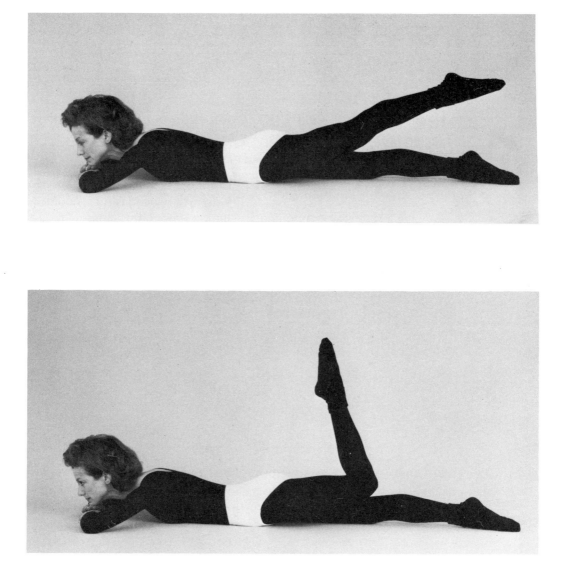

7

Bicycle

1. Lie on your back. Bend your left leg and place your hands below the knee. Extend your right leg forward, foot pointed and raised slightly off the floor.

2. Keeping a rhythmic tempo, alternate drawing one knee to your chest as you extend the other leg forward. Keep your breathing steady, repeating 12 times on each leg. Rest by hugging both knees to your chest for 6 slow counts.

Repetition: Three complete sets

If you want to challenge yourself further, try this same exercise with your head and shoulders lifted off the floor. Either way, it's important that you concentrate on keeping your abdominal muscles pulled in and the extended leg low.

(Tip) Don't succumb to advertising hype that offers miracle cures for cellulite. They don't exist. But do try to drink lots of water, at least eight glasses a day are recommended to help flush out impurities from the system.

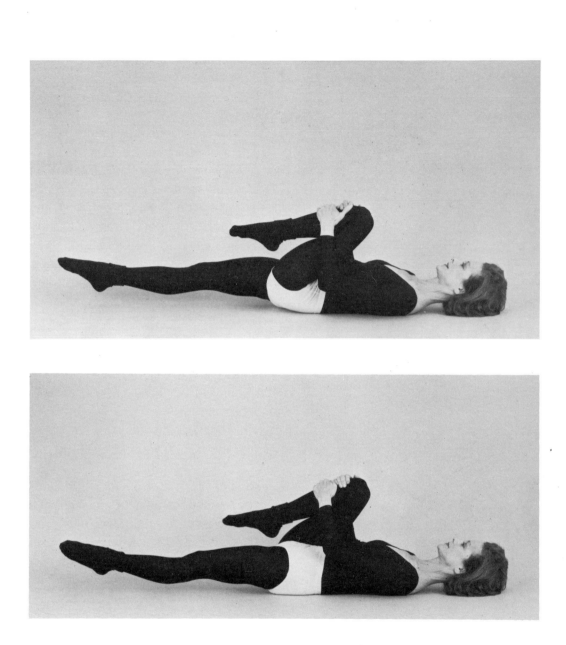

8

PRESCRIPTION FOR WOMEN WHO ARE ON THEIR FEET

Your exercise needs are unique and important to address if your work keeps you on your feet for the greater part of your day. That's why the routine designed for you specifically zeros in on developing strength and flexibility in the foot and leg as well as improving circulation to these areas.

Women who stand a great deal—nurses, saleswomen, flight attendants, dental technicians, etc. must all pay special attention to the health of their feet and legs. Legs and feet which are "unhappy" because of bad circulation, weak muscles, poor balance or constricting shoes can cause not only discomfort but backaches, neck pain and an all-over feeling of fatigue. Let's face it, when your legs and feet are tired and unhappy, the rest of you can't feel all that great.

Additionally, the woman who stands for extended periods without moving is at a greater disadvantage than the one who stands but is more active. When you stand in place for a prolonged period, your leg muscles cannot do their pumping action through the veins. That's how fluid collects. (Swollen ankles are caused by an accumulation of fluid in the bottom of the legs.) For this reason, I generally suggest to my clients who primarily stand in place for several hours to walk wherever or whenever possible. This is important, since the chief way that blood comes uphill from the lower extremities is by action of the muscles on the veins. If the muscles are not exercised every day to some degree, your circulation will inevitably suffer. Remember, circulation is improved by motion. You don't have to climb mountains or run marathons, just move at your own comfortable pace, as much as possible.

One of my clients, a saleswoman at a prestigious Manhattan jewellery store, claims that at the end of her day, her feet "cry" out for help. I've recommended that she massage them when she arrives home after work in order to activate the circulation and alleviate some of the fatigue. Alcohol rubs can be stimulating and refreshing too. Or, for truly exhausted feet, you might try a ten-minute soak in warm water and Epsom salts. Because your feet are so far away from your heart, foot circulation must really be worked on.

When resting, it's a good idea to raise your feet, not just off the floor but higher than your heart. This is an effective way to revitalize circulation in your legs and relax tired, stood-on feet. Also, it will help to prevent, or relieve, varicose veins. Try, if possible, to elevate your feet at least twice a day for three or four minutes. A simple way to do this is to lie on the floor with your head in your hands and your feet raised and propped against a wall. Just make certain to keep your lower back flat and your buttocks at least ten inches from the wall.

Using a slant board is a great way to treat your legs and feet to the benefits of elevation. Just lying down on one can be marvelously therapeutic if you've been standing all day. You don't even have to exercise on it, just lie there and relax. In fact, it's the ideal time to practise the deep-breathing exercise I've included in the relaxation segment in Chapter 6. Not only will your legs and feet thank you for time spent on the slant board, but your hair and skin will benefit as well. That's because elevating your feet higher than your heart causes your blood flow to reverse, sending vital nutrients to your skin and scalp.

Another client, a department store executive, claims that ten minutes on her slant board refreshes and revives her more than a catnap for nonstop evenings on the town. Her slant-board ritual includes the removal of her make-up first, followed by the application of a vitalizing skin mask. The mask performs its magic while soothing music and dim lighting add to the calming effect.

What might you use in lieu of a regulation slant board? Years ago, I discovered that lying on top of my ironing board (slanted of course) could do as well. And how pleasant to use it for beautifying instead of ironing!

Simply prop up the narrow end, resting it approximately eighteen inches off the floor, on something that will allow for maximum support. My bed is the ideal height. In addition, I usually place a pillow under my neck and head for cushioning and comfort. (Admittedly, I have been known to nod off for a few minutes on occasion.) When I'm more energetic, I might do a few stretching exercises but nothing too taxing or invigorating.

I think you will find that the benefits of resting on a slant board are many. Not only will it stimulate and improve leg circulation, but lying there will ease the back-muscle fatigue that so often results from being on one's feet continually. In fact, if your back is particularly tired, rest for a while with your knees bent and the soles of your feet flat on the board. You might even try practicing the basic pelvic tilt exercise to strengthen the back muscles and ease pain and fatigue as well. Simply tilt your pelvis up as you contract your abdominals and press your spine against the board. Hold the contraction for six slow counts, making sure no space exists between the board and your back. Then relax the contraction. In order to derive maximum benefit from the tilt, exhale while pulling in your abdominals and inhale when you release. A final word about using a slant board of any kind. When you're ready to get off the board, make certain to lift yourself slowly in order to avoid dizziness.

In talking with orthopaedists and chiropodists, I find all agree that wearing the right shoes contributes to the health of one's feet and legs. But what are the "right" shoes? Certainly not an overly high heel. They make standing for any length of time painful, walking exhausting, and running impossible. High heels throw you off balance. To see what I mean, strip down in front of a full-length mirror and watch yourself walk across the room in high heels. The knee must bend, the lumbar region creates an extra-high arch, the neck cranes and the head is held badly. High heels also thwart the motion of the foot from going through its shock-absorbing action. This affects the joints all the way up the leg and into your back, jarring your entire body.

Now, I'm not suggesting that you wear sneakers to the theater or a gala. For short periods of time, at work or social occasions, high heels are fine. But for walking considerable distances, they're definitely not recommended footwear. Your feet may protest by developing bunions, corns and hammertoes. Select a more comfortable low-heeled shoe, one that fits snugly in the heel area and loosely enough for the toes to wiggle. If your shoe is too narrow in the toe space, your foot muscles will tense, followed by your leg muscles and the muscles in your back as well. So, too, shoe heels that fit incorrectly cause your ankles to wobble, affecting your knees, hips joints and neck. Opt for leather soles and shoes. Leather is soft, flexible, and allows the foot to breathe.

The exercises in this segment are tailored to strengthen the legs and feet while simultaneously increasing circulation. You may also wish to incorporate some of the back strengthening movements that have been included in Chapter 9. If you spend a great deal of time on your feet, you probably experience some degree of lower back discomfort or fatigue. To correct this, it is important that your back and abdominals are as strong and resilient.

Whenever you can, punctuate your daily activities with some simple foot exercises such as an occasional flexing and pointing sequence or ankle rotations. When flexing the foot, really try to press the heel forward so that you feel the stretch all the way to your calf. While standing and talking on the telephone, for example, rise to your toes, then lower your heels in order to relieve rigidity in the ankles and the longitudinal arch. Or, to stretch the tendons on the top of the foot, sit with your bare feet on the floor and try to pick up a pencil or marble with your toes.

Your feet are your friends and they carry a heavy load. When your feet hurt . . . you hurt. Bound by stockings or tights and stuffed into sweaty shoes all day, feet are the most trod-upon and forgotten part of the body. Start treating them right today. Remember, feet have feelings too.

PRESCRIPTION FOR WOMEN WHO ARE ON THEIR FEET

1

Pulse Plié

1. Stand with your feet shoulder-width apart and turned out. Rest your hands on your waist.

2. Bend your knees over your feet, keeping your shoulders in line with your hips. In this position, gently pulse your knees down 6 times, keeping your buttocks tucked under and your abdominal muscles pulled in. Then straighten your legs to the original position.

Repetition: Three sets

(Tip) Ninety percent of people have feet of slightly different lengths. If you are among them, fit the longer foot; use tongue or heel pads on the other foot to snug up the heel or toe.

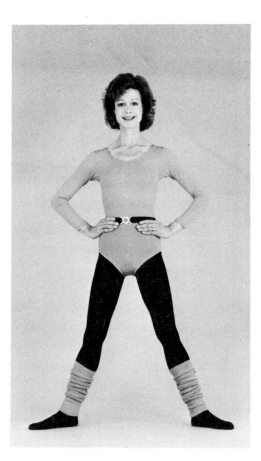

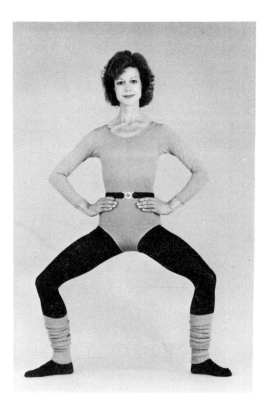

2

Quadriceps Strengthener

1. Sit with your right foot on the floor and the knee close to your body. Clasp your hands below the knee. Extend your left leg in front, foot flexed and raised slightly off of the floor.

2. Keeping your abdominal muscles contracted, lift, then lower, the leg within a few inches of the floor.

Exhale with each lift. Repeat 8 times slowly, then 8 times double time. Repeat on the right leg.

Repetition: Two sets on each leg

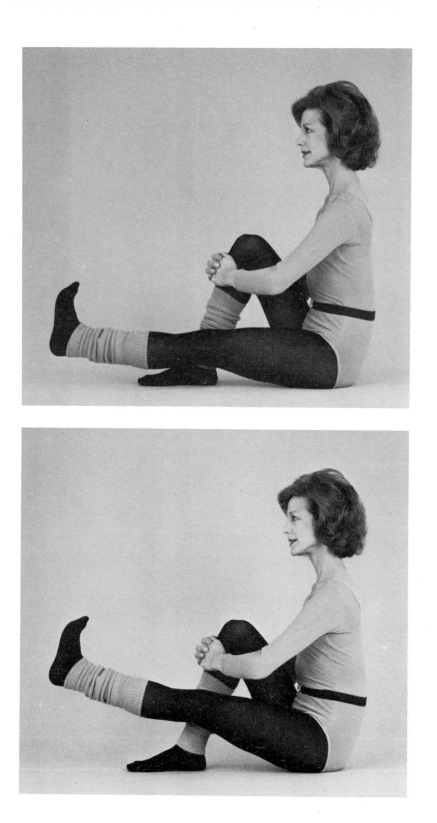

3

Inner Thigh Firmer

1. Lie on your back, feet raised, with your right foot crossed over your left, knees wide apart. Rest your hands under your buttocks to support your lower back, abdominal muscles contracted.

2. Exhale your breath as you extend your legs out to the sides, abdominal muscles contracted. Then inhale and bend your legs, crossing the left foot over the right. Repeat 16 times. Release by hugging both knees to your chest for the count of 4.

Repetition: Two sets

(Tip) Toenail-snip tip. Trim them wet, not dry. There's less nail trauma, less cracking.

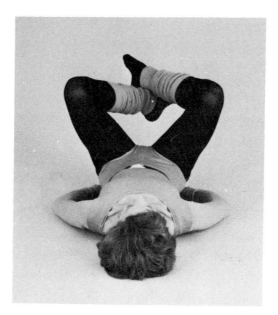

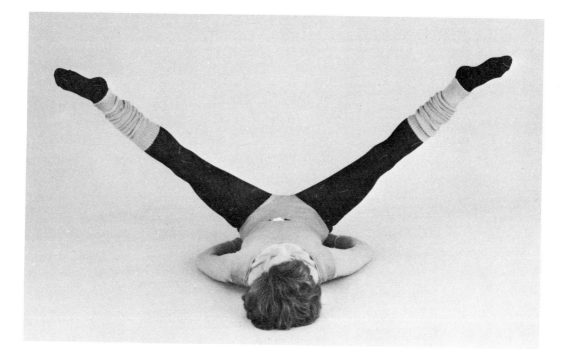

4

The Windmill

1. Lie on your back. Extend your right leg toward the ceiling and place your hands near the calf. Extend your left leg in front, foot pointed and raised slightly off of the floor.

2. Release your grip on your right leg and lower it practically to the floor as you simultaneously ease your left leg toward your body. Rhythmically change hands from one leg to the other as you keep your breathing relaxed and steady. Repeat 10 times on each leg. Release by hugging your knees to your chest for a count of 5.

Repetition: Two sets

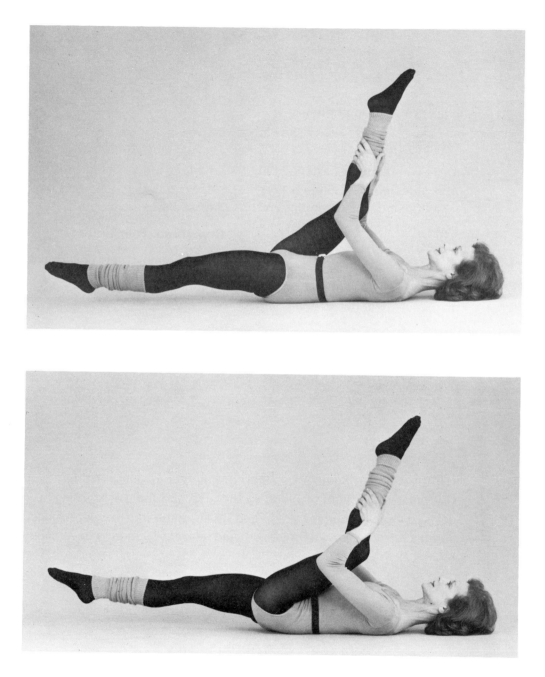

5

Hamstring Strengthener

1. Sit with your legs extended in front, toes pointed. Stretch your torso forward from your hips and place your hands on or near your ankles.

2. Keeping your upper body lengthened, flex your feet as hard as you can without straining and hold for 8 slow counts, breathing steady and deep. Release your grip and shake out your legs.

Repetition: Four times

If the stretch is too challenging, try it with slightly bent knees.

(Tip) If you've suffered a leg strain or pull, you require cold, not heat; cold inhibits the flow of blood to the area and reduces swelling. The quickest route to soothing strains and sprains starts with the four-pronged approach—rest, ice, compression and elevation, more conveniently known as RICE.

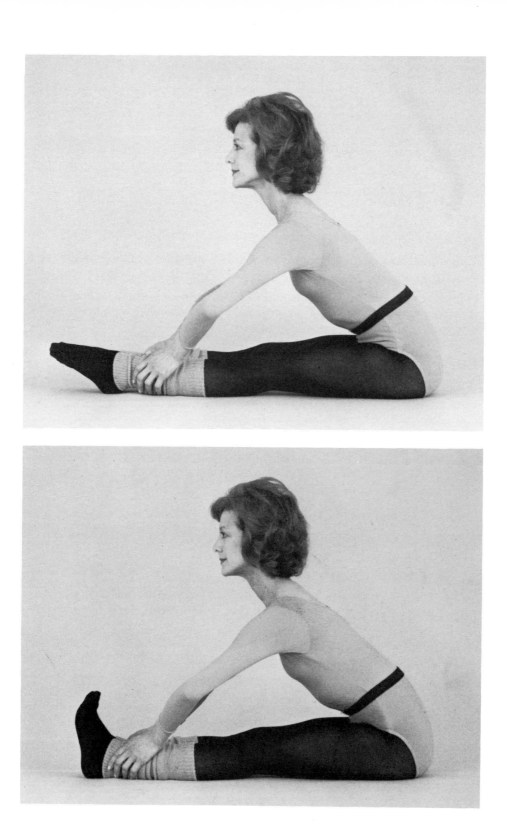

6

Foot Rotation

1. Lie on your back with your arms relaxed at your sides. Place your left foot on the floor and extend your right leg up, foot pointed.

2. Keeping the leg stationary, rotate your foot clockwise 8 times, then reverse direction. Repeat on the left foot.

Repetition: Two complete sets on each foot

The foot rotation is an exercise that you can easily insert into your schedule, while seated at your breakfast table or desk, in an aeroplane or taxi, etc. It not only strengthens the ankle but stimulates circulation as well.

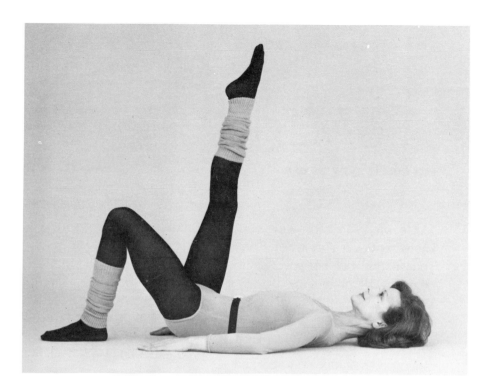

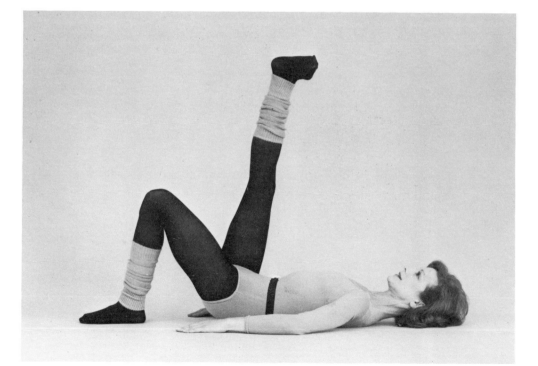

7

Leg Lift/Tummy Sleeker

1. Lie on your back with your knees bent over your waist. Place your hands behind your head, elbows wide open.

2. Contract your abdominal muscles and lift your head and shoulders off the floor. Simultaneously straighten your legs and bring your elbows forward. Hold for 2 counts, then release to the original position. Repeat 12 times. Hug your knees to your chest for 6 counts. Exhale on the lift and inhale on the release.

Repetition: Three sets

With any sit-up or "crunch" movement, roll your head slowly from side to side between sets if you experience any neck fatigue. The trick is to train your abdominals to do the work, not your neck.

(Tip) For support hose to be effective, the pressure should be strongest around the ankles and decrease as it goes up the calf.

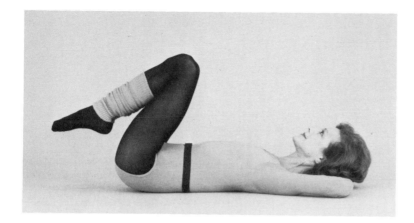

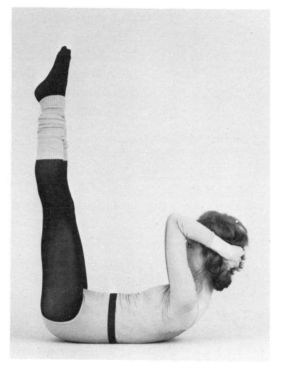

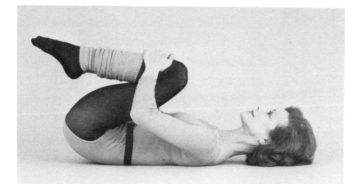

151

9

PRESCRIPTION FOR WOMEN WHO SLUMP AND SLOUCH

Hunching over a desk, drawing board or kitchen table or peering at a computer screen from nine to five can put the most finely toned body into a posture predicament. The result: round shoulders, a drooping chest, stiff neck and strained upper-back muscles. Musclewise, there's a dual dilemma at play. First, the back muscles that keep shoulders "square" become too weak from slouching to do the job well; at the same time, the opposing muscles in the chest area tighten up and resist the back muscles.

Experts agree that long hours spent sitting incorrectly stresses the spine and can lead to various orthopaedic problems—most commonly, back pain, from mild to severe. Studies indicate, however, that people with strong back and abdominal muscles are much less likely to develop problems related to prolonged sitting than those with muscles in poor condition. That's why this section accents exercises that will improve your back's strength and suppleness while at the same time increasing abdominal control and tone. When you strengthen the stress-prone upper and lower back muscles, they become less vulnerable to stiffness-causing pressures. The stronger the muscles, the more easily they can absorb tension. For that reason, activities such as swimming and cross-country skiing are very effective. They use, and strengthen, the upper body.

Many members of the "slumped and slouched" set pay scant attention to the highly unhealthy position in which they spend the better part of a day. You're probably seated as you read these words. Assess your posture. Are you lifted and thus lengthening your body? Chances are good that you are tilted forward, with your back flexed, abdomen extended, neck curved. While sitting, most women fail to use their abdominal or extensor (located along the back) muscles to support their spine. This places pressure on the intervertebral disks, the layers of fibrous tissue located between the vertebrae. This pressure may push the disks against the nerves of the spine, which can cause considerable discomfort. Sitting with the back flexed also stresses and tightens the ligaments between the vertebrae. In time, these ligaments become fatigued and develop microtears, which cause the stiffness and discomfort many women experience when they stand up and try to straighten their backs. By learning to lift your ribs away from your hips (seated and standing) you expand your abdominal cavity, allowing for better breathing and uncramped internal organs. Keep this lifted image in mind as you practice the movements in this section.

One of my clients, a concert pianist, originally consulted with me because of pain she was experiencing in the muscles of her neck, shoulders and upper back. Her condition was provoked by slumping forward for hours on end at the keyboard. In her particular case, the problem was further aggravated by stress and tension. Needless to say, tension, caused by work or home-related problems can block the effects of even the most beneficial exercise program. By designing a regimen for this woman that concentrated on strengthening her upper back muscles, I enabled her to better manage the physical demands of her profession.

Although it is difficult to concentrate on your alignment throughout the day, understanding the principles of correct seated posture can be very beneficial. When you are seated, your spine should be in the same position as when you stand, forming three natural curves: cervical (neck), thoracic (chest), and lumbar (lower back). In order to sit correctly you must lift the chest by extending the muscles of the back; compress the abdominal muscles, which creates pressure inside of the abdominal cavity and supports the spine. Your shoulders should be straight and relaxed, ears in line with your hips. Again I underscore the importance of not crossing your legs, which further stresses the spine and promotes circulatory problems as well. Feet should be planted firmly on the floor. When standing, look for three problem areas: rounded shoulders, swayed lower back, hyperextended (locked) knees. The cure: practise standing, sitting, walking as if you have a string pulling you up from the top of your head. The key words to remember are *lift and lengthen.*

I truly believe that one of the most effective exercises for strengthening the abdominal muscles is the pelvic tilt. It's the exercise I probably emphasize most in my classes. By developing the ability to execute the tilt with ease, you will not only strengthen your back but you will also develop the necessary control to exercise with proper alignment, energy and ease.

In my teaching experience, I have found that most women do not understand the extreme importance of starting with a good pelvic tilt and maintaining it while doing curl-ups, sit-ups, crunches or abdominal strengthening movements of any kind. If you neglect to tilt *first,* the abdominals will push forward, placing pressure on your lower back. When practising the exercises in this section, as well as throughout the book, make a supreme effort to give adequate emphasis to proper abdominal control coupled with correct breathing. When you inhale, your abdominal muscles naturally stretch and expand under the pressure of the air in your lungs. It is thus self-defeating to attempt to contract against this pressure. That's why the exhalation should always accompany the contraction. It will make a significant difference as to the benefits you derive from the movements.

Using weights can be effective for developing greater upper-back strength. In class, I generally recommend three- to five-pound weights, which gets the job done without causing strain for most women. If, however, that seems excessive, you might opt for less. Should you not have a pair of weights or dumbbells to work with, improvise by using something of comparable weight. I've found that for a lighter weight, two full cylindrical cartons of salt are inexpensive, nonbreakable and easy to grasp. Make certain that whenever you do work with weights you pay special attention to correct breath control. Always exhale on the exertion. That's truly essential, or you will strain unnecessarily. It is important also that you refrain from locking your elbows when using weights. Try to keep them slightly "soft." As for working with weights while standing, it's essential to tuck your buttocks under and avoid locking your knees. For beginners in particular, I generally advise that weight work be done lying on one's back with knees bent, since it is easier to maintain the pelvic tilt in that position.

Another exercise that is worthwhile as a spine straightener and strengthener and can be done during the course of your day, is the following: With your feet hip-width apart, lean back against a wall, full-length mirror or door frame. Bend your knees and squat, as if you were sitting on a chair, your back and head against the wall. Use your abdominals to really flatten your lower spine against the wall. With your arms extended in front at chest level, slide up and down several times maintaining the pelvic tilt. In addition to strengthening your spine and abdominals, the bonus from this exercise will be stronger quadriceps as well.

Strong quadriceps and well-stretched hamstrings are important to back health. Women with tight hamstring muscles tend to tilt the base of the pelvis back which leads to an exaggerated lumbar curve (swayback). If yours need stretching, you might wish to tag on to this regimen some of the hamstring exercises from other sections as well. One that is particularly worthwhile is the hamstring strengthener in the previous chapter. As for strengthening the quadriceps, controlled knee bends (pliés) particularly with the feet parallel and the cycling exercise are both recommended.

As your abdominal muscles become stronger from this routine, they will act as a greater support for your spine. Remember, the two work in tandem. Again, I must underscore the importance of breathing properly. Build up to the suggested repetitions slowly if you initially find the numbers too challenging. Above all, try to regularly incorporate some, or all, of these conditioning exercises into your personal workout plan. By priming your muscles to *lift* and *lengthen,* you'll sit and stand taller, feel stronger and radiate a confident, approachable image.

PRESCRIPTION FOR THE WOMAN WHO SLUMPS AND SLOUCHES

1

Overhead Reach

1. Sit tall with your legs extended to the sides, toes pointed. Extend your arms up, chin slightly raised.

2. Alternating arms, stretch first with the right, then with the left, trying to reach higher and higher with each stretch. Repeat 8 times on each side. Lower your head and round your back. With your palms on the floor and elbows bent, hold the stretch for 4 counts, keeping your breathing normal. Then uncurl, beginning at the base of your spine and repeat the sequence.

Repetition: Twice

(Tip) A good way to release the pressure on your back while you sit at a desk or table is to put a telephone book on the floor and rest one foot on it. This will tilt your pelvis back and flatten the lumbar curve.

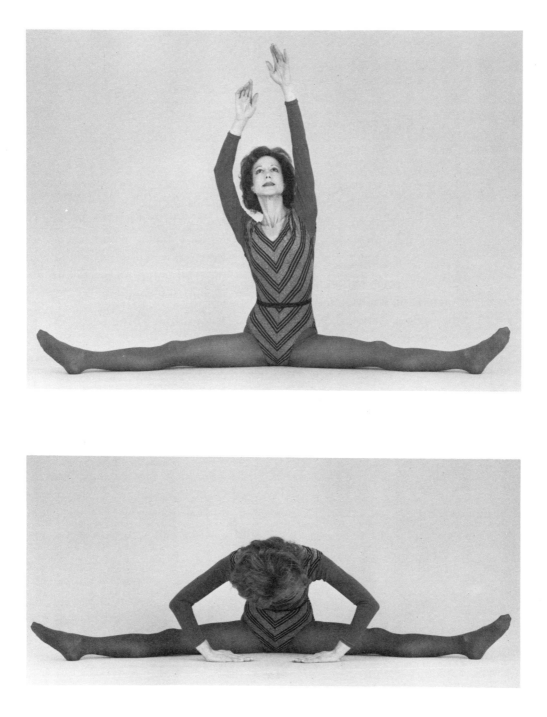

2

Upper Back Strengthener

1. Lie on your back with your knees bent, feet parallel and hip-width apart. Hold a three-pound weight in your extended arms, palms facing out.

2. With your abdominals contracted and your spine flat against the floor, slowly release the weight back until it practically touches the floor. Lift it several inches, then release it again, without touching the floor. Repeat 12 times, exhaling with each lowering motion. Lift your arms up to the original position before repeating the sequence.

Repetition: Three sets

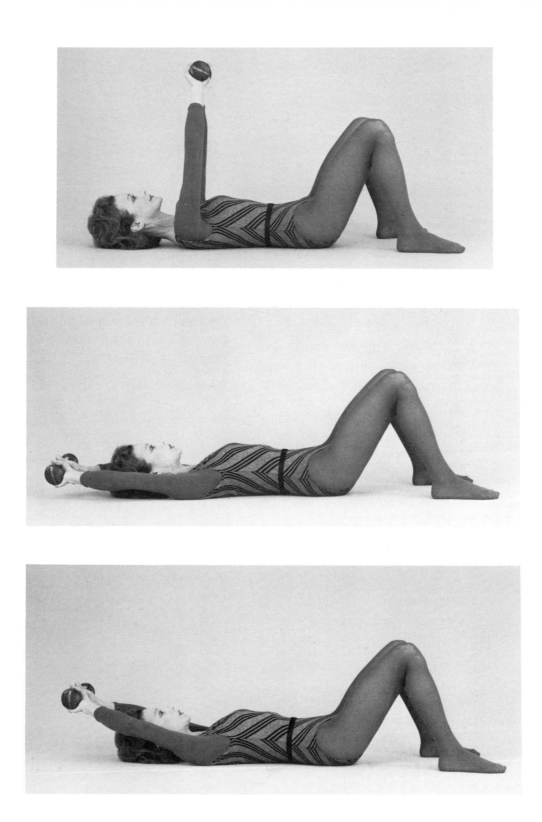

3

Leg Up Crunch

1. Lie on your back with your left knee bent, foot resting on the floor. Place your right leg on your left thigh and your hands behind your head, elbows wide open.

2. Contract your abdominals and exhale as you lift your head and upper back off the floor. Keep your elbows wide open and your chin lifted. Release just slightly, then lift again. Repeat this small, upward pulsing motion 20 times, exhaling with each lift. Roll down to the floor, and before repeating with the left leg extended, relax by rolling your head slowly from side to side.

Repetition: Two complete sets

(Tip) Proper desk height for good alignment: when you bend your elbow, the desk top should be approximately one inch above the point of your elbow; a little bit lower for typing and computer tables.

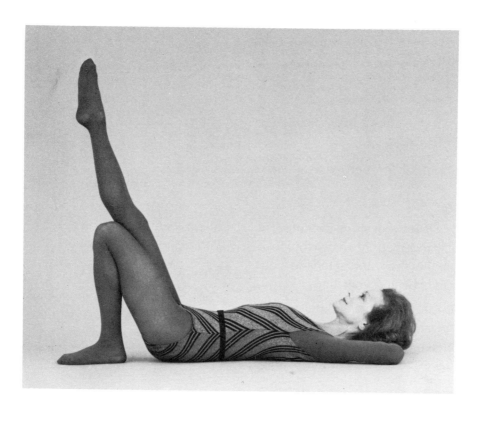

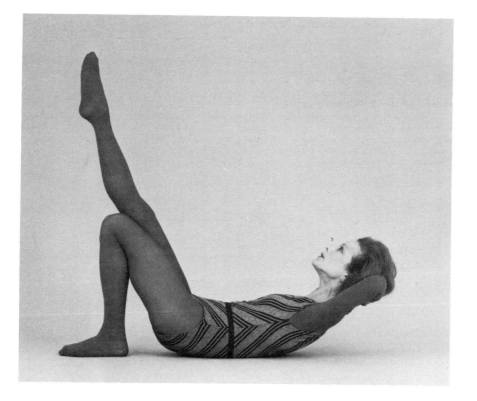

4

Shoulder Strengthener

1. Lie on your stomach with your legs together. Rest your forehead on the floor and interlace your hands behind your body.

2. Lift your arms and pulse them upward 10 times, feeling the stretch between your shoulder blades. Release them to the origi-nal position. Accompany each lift with a short exhalation.

Repetition: Three sets

If you contract your buttock mus-cles, you will derive a bonus ton-ing from this exercise.

***

(Tip) A heavy shoulder bag pulls the body off center. Switch the bag frequently from one shoulder to the other so that one side is not over-stressed.

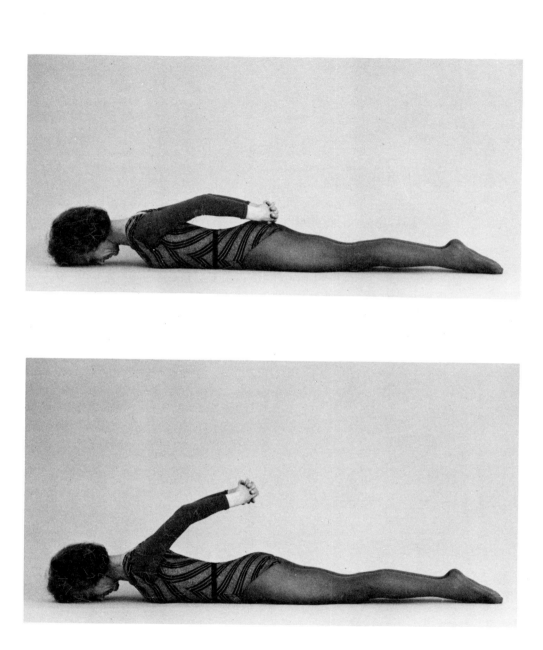

5

Roll Back

1. Sit upright with your knees bent. Place your feet hip-width apart and parallel on the floor. Interlace your hands behind your head, elbows wide apart.

2. Contract your abdominal muscles first. Then exhale as you slowly roll back, shoulders rounded, elbows forward. Stop before your waist touches the floor. Inhale and slowly lift to the original straight-back position. Take 3 counts to roll back and 3 to lift. Repeat 12 times. To relax between sets, stretch forward from your hips and reach for your toes, knees slightly bent.

Repetition: Three sets

(Tip) Keep your work as close to eye level as possible in order not to distort your alignment or cause neck strain.

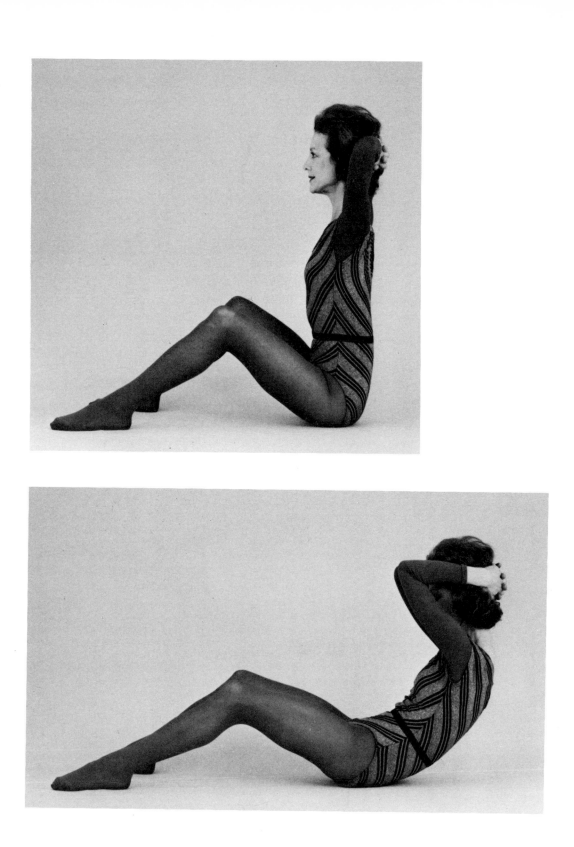

6

Pelvic Tilt Slide

1. Lie on your back with your knees bent and your feet placed comfortably apart on the floor. Place your hands behind your head or relax them at your sides.

2. Contract your abdominal muscles and press the small of your back into the floor. Slowly slide your legs forward, trying to straighten them while maintaining the tilt. Stop at the point when you are no longer able to keep your spine flat. Try to time a slow exhalation to the sliding motion.

Repetition: Six times

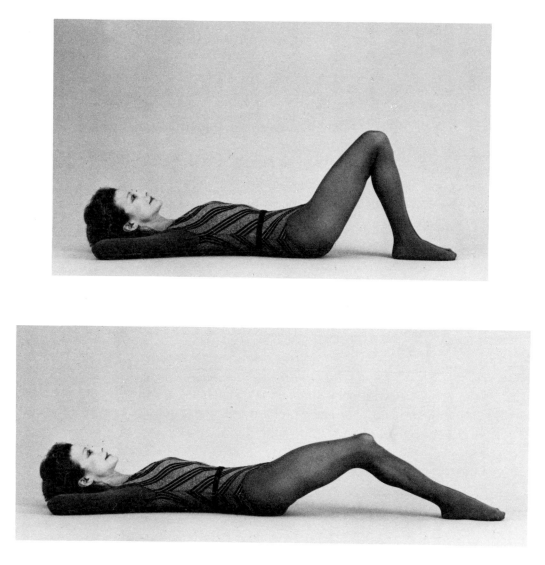

7

Backup

1. Begin on your forearms and knees. Rest your forehead on top of your interlaced hands.

2. Contract your abdominal muscles as you exhale. At the same time, slowly round your back beginning at the base of your spine. Hold 2 slow counts, then release to the original position without letting your back arch.

Repetition: Eight times

Make an effort to really pull your lower abdominal muscles in. In addition to strengthening the spine, this exercise relaxes it as well.

(**Tip**) To avoid neck strain, don't clutch the telephone between your shoulder and your ear. Purchase a phone cradle that eases strain and frees up your hands to do other tasks.

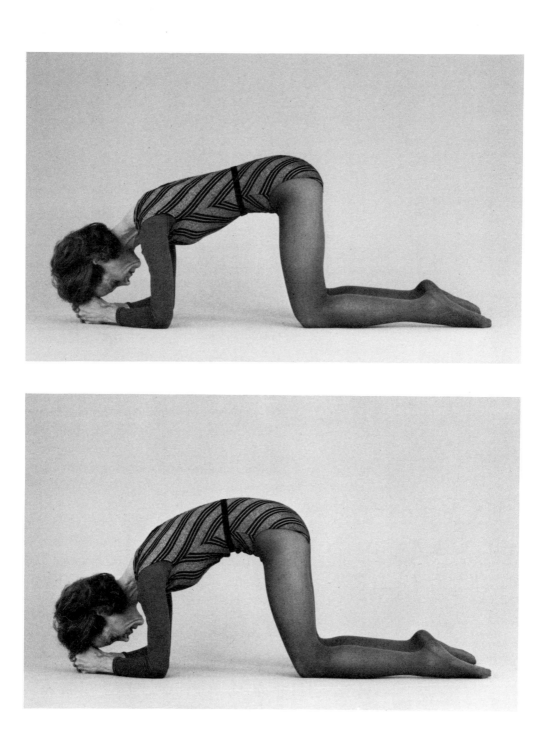

10

PRESCRIPTION
FOR WOMEN
WHO TRAVEL

Abandoning your fitness programme need not be the consequence of frequent business travel. The woman who travels extensively can take her programme on the road. Today, there are a multitude of fitness options available. They can be as simple as the in-seat movements prescribed in the airline magazines, stretching in the bath or shower, swimming, running, or even partaking in a class at a nearby fitness centre or dance studio.

Business travel formerly meant periods of enforced and often unwelcome leisure. Fortunately, this is no longer the case. Inspired by fitness "mania," hotels, health clubs and even the airlines are providing travellers with ready access to gym facilities, special programmes and even nutritionally inspired meals such as the one designed by the American Heart Association. Studies confirm that the public has responded very favourably. Women who travel for business are proving more than ever before that they will go out of their way to stay at a hotel that offers facilities of one kind or another . . . a pool for swimming laps, an indoor track or a room filled with standard weight equipment.

Aeroplanes may be the fastest way to get there, but don't be surprised if you arrive feeling exhausted, irritable, disoriented and wishing you were at home in your own bed. Long flights can truly play havoc with the body. That's why it's so important to punctuate your in-flight time with some discreet dekinking exercises. They will boost circulation and reduce the stiffness and tension that inevitably set in during extended flights. I make it a habit to get up frequently from my seat (I always reserve one on the aisle) and walk the length of the plane. Or I make an excuse to stretch for something in the overhead compartment. Many of the in-chair movements included in the office segment in Section I can be practised in your plane seat as well. They will activate your blood flow and relax tight muscles. Keeping stiffness at bay makes all the difference as to how you will feel once you arrive at your final destination.

When I began traveling extensively for business, I realized I did not have to be held captive to airline food. With just a bit of planning ahead, you can order a special meal. This can be done when you make your reservation or, should you forget to do so, by calling the airline twenty-four hours in advance. I have eliminated red meat from my diet so I select from the vegetarian, seafood or fruit plate. I pre-order these meals even when I fly first class. (First-class airline meals tend to be loaded with high-fat fare.) When you board the plane, make certain to alert the flight attendant to your seat location and to which meal you pre-ordered. Sometimes, particularly if I'm travelling to the West Coast or to Europe, I pack a favourite sandwich, which often turns out to be white meat turkey and cos lettuce (with mustard) on crusty French bread. In my personal CARE package I include some fresh fruit as well as several mini boxes of raisins, which satisfy my sweet tooth and keeps my energy level up. I make certain to drink lots of water or soda water (my exercise comes from frequent visits to the lavatory) and I avoid drinking alcoholic beverages as well as those containing caffeine.

No woman should desert her fitness regime when she's away from her usual workout environment. According to some sports-medicine pros, your body begins to get less fit within as little as seventy-two hours. Now that's a depressing thought! After ten to fourteen inactive days, fitness considerably diminishes as a result of the loss of muscle resilience.

When you travel, your objective should not be to put your body to the test, but instead to try to *maintain* its fitness level. Your goals should be realistic and manageable. Even if you do some exercise, be it relaxing yoga postures or light swimming, it's better than doing nothing at all and returning home looking worse than your abused baggage.

I think planning a personal exercise timetable is particularly important when you travel, since your days can become overbooked and disrupted. For me, it's helpful to schedule exercise as I do other appointments. If I miss one day, I make an extra effort to work out the next, otherwise I might start skipping regularly and get out of the "exercise habit." Once you break the habit, it's easier not to exercise.

I generally find my hotel room is a convenient place in which to work out, even if space is somewhat limited. Should the carpet lack padding, or be anything less than inviting, I then request an additional blanket from housekeeping to cover my workout area. Sometimes, I check the television schedule the night before so that I can awaken in time to stretch with the local guru. This can be fun. When I remain in one location for an extended period of time, I try to sample a class at a recommended dance or yoga studio. Many studios, or even the YWCA, allow you to pay by the class.

Running is also part of my personal fitness routine, so I generally try to stay at a hotel that accommodates my needs with safe and pleasant running routes nearby. Oftentimes, this means staying at a hotel near a park or marina. I've discovered that when I am travelling alone, running first thing in the morning is a wonderful way for me to see the sights and experience a new environment. Many hotels even offer walking maps or guides.

The in-hotel room programme that follows is one that respects the fact that your space is probably quite limited. Lunges, leg swings and movements that require an expansive area have been totally eliminated from this segment. Instead, you will find the routine contained and manageable. If, however, you feel less than enthusiastic about lying on the floor, many of the exercises can be done on the bed. Should this be your choice, you might want to request a bedboard from housekeeping (I generally do) to assure firmness and support. In addition, you can extend the routine by tagging on some of the in-bed stretches I've included in Section I of the book. Or, should you be fortunate enough to be staying in the presidential suite, or something equally spacious, feel free to incorporate a selection of your favourite less contained movements from other sections of this book as well.

You can, with a bit of thought and effort, turn business travel into a healthy, positive experience. It can mean time out for you . . . a time for some special pampering. After all, who gets the sheets changed at home every day or chocolates placed on her pillow nightly?

1

Inner Thigh Slimmer

1. Sit tall with the soles of your feet together, hands resting on your feet.

2. Round your back and bend your elbows in front of your legs. Keeping your knees low and your head relaxed, gently press your body toward the floor 12 times exhaling with each downward motion. Uncurl beginning at the base of your spine until your back is straight and your knees release.

Repetition: Three sets

(Tip) Try to adapt to the time frame of your destination. If local time is noon and your biological clock says 5 P.M. it's best to stay awake until the locals go to bed. You'll adjust more rapidly.

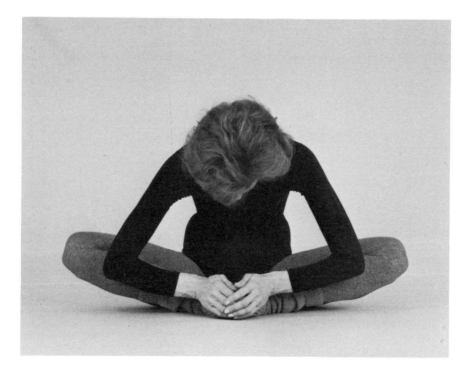

2

Crossed Ankle Thigh Stretch

1. Lie on your back with your hands behind your head. Lift your feet and cross them at the ankles, knees as wide apart as possible.

2. Keeping your feet crossed, exhale and extend your legs up until they are straight. Bend them to the open-knee position, feeling a good stretch on the inner thigh. Repeat 20 times.

Repetition: Three sets

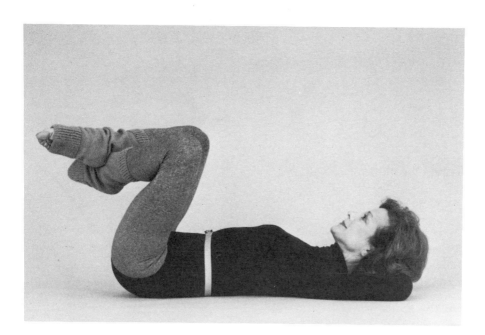

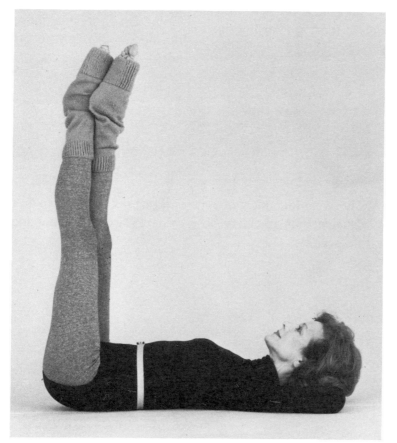

3

Travel Crunch

1. Lie on your back with your legs extended, knees slightly bent over your waist. Place your hands behind your head, elbows wide open.

2. Contract your abdominal muscles and lift your head and shoulders off the floor, keeping the elbows wide apart. Lower slightly but do not touch the floor. Repeat the lift-release motion 12 times exhaling with each lift. Lower your legs and body and hug your knees to your chest for 4 counts.

Repetition: Three sets

Train your abdominal muscles to do the work, not your arms or neck.

(Tip) Always wear identification when jogging out of town. In an emergency, valuable time could be lost trying to ascertain your identity, medical history, etc.

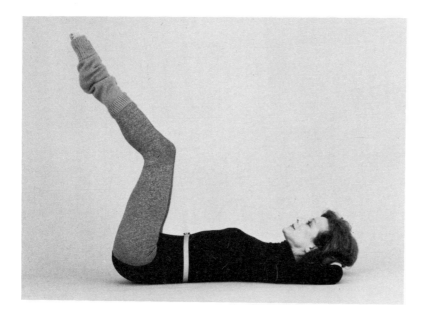

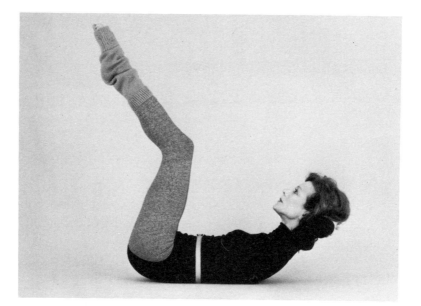

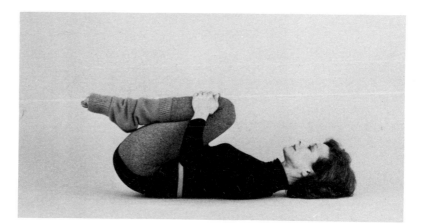

4

Leg Up/Buttock Lift

1. Lie on your back with your hands behind your head. Bend your left knee and place the foot on the floor. Extend your right leg up, foot pointed.

2. Contract your abdominal muscles and tilt your pelvis as you raise your buttocks off the floor. Do not lift your waist. In this contracted position, pulse upward 12 times with small, controlled "squeezes" (squeeze-release). Roll down to the floor and lower your leg. Repeat with the left leg extended. With each squeeze, exhale your breath.

Repetition: Two sets on each leg

(Tip) Altitude changes demand that you give your body time to adjust; modify your workouts. Remember, too, the risk of dehydration is intensified at high altitudes.

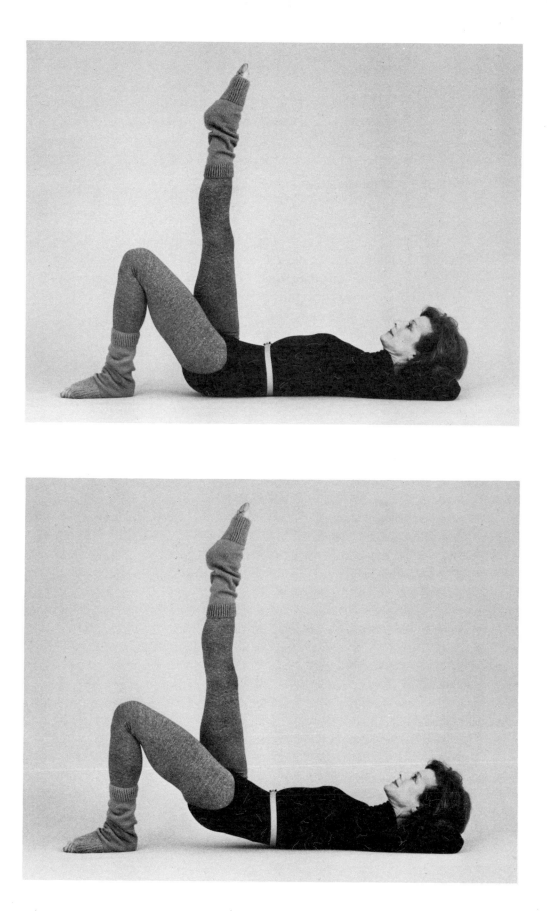

5

Thigh Tightener

1. Sit with your left knee bent parallel to the floor, foot close to your body. Bend your right knee and place your hands near the ankle (or higher up if it's more comfortable). Point your right foot and rest your toes on the floor.

2. Exhale as you extend your leg forward, then bend it. Keep your abdominal muscles tucked in. Repeat 12 times on each leg, trying to keep your upper body lifted and lengthened.

Repetition: Three sets

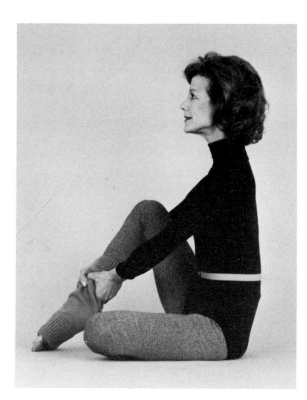

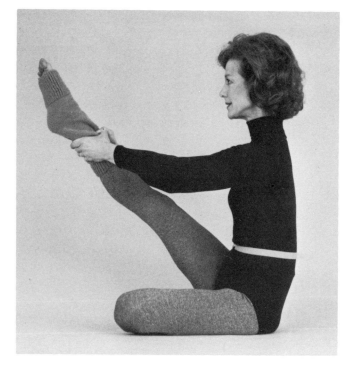

6

Waist Twister

1. Sit with your ankles crossed and your hands interlaced behind your head, elbows wide open to the sides.

2. Twist your upper body from your waist, lowering your right elbow to your left knee. Keep the left elbow raised as high as possible. Return to a lifted centre position, then twist to the right. Exhale on the twist and inhale on the lift.

Remember, the lift is as important as the twist.

Repetition: Twelve times to each side

(Tip) Allow roughly one day per each time zone crossed to adjust to the new environment. For the first few days, reduce the intensity and duration of your regular workout.

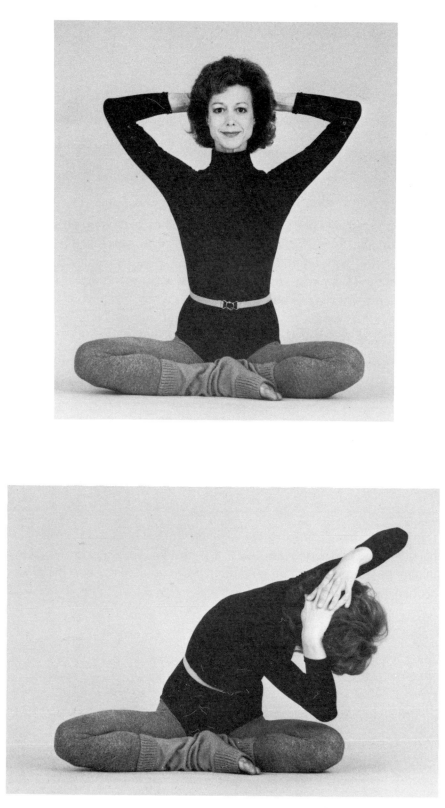

7

Turn Around

1. Sit with your left knee bent and resting on the floor. Cross your right foot over your left thigh and rest it on the floor. Rest your left heel against your right buttock, arms relaxed.

2. Turn your upper body from the waist to your left. Place your right hand on your right heel and your left hand on the floor behind you. Look over your left shoulder. Hold this position for a slow count of 30 pulling up through your torso in order to really feel the stretch. Keep your breathing natural and relaxed. Repeat the twist to your right.

Repetition: Once on each side

(Tip) Plastic bags from the dry cleaner work wonders for clothes on hangers. The air trapped inside acts as a cushion and keeps creasing to a minimum. Your clothes can go directly from your suitcase to the closet, no hanger changes necessary.

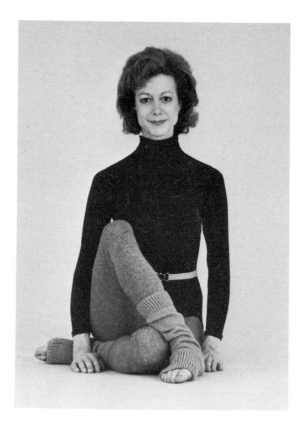

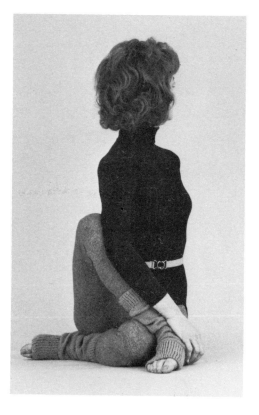

GLOSSARY

It is important that you understand the following movement terms frequently used throughout this book:

CONTRACTION: A tightening of the muscle(s). Throughout, you will be reminded to "contract" or "tighten" your abdominal and buttock muscles.

PULSE: A small, controlled movement that can be done upward, downward or laterally. A pulse is less staccato than a bounce, which tends to be more abrupt and jerky.

EXTENSION: Stretching or straightening the arm or leg at any angle to the body.

FLEX: This refers to the position of the foot. When you flex your foot, your toes are pulled back toward your leg and your heel is pressed forward. Flexing is the opposite of pointing, in which the toes are pushed forward and downward, thus elongating the line of the leg.

GRIP: To tighten or contract (i.e., the buttocks or abdominals).

PLIÉ: With feet either parallel or turned out, a bending of the knees over the feet.

TILT: The motion in which the pelvis is lifted.

TUCK: The position in which the abdominals are "scooped in" or the buttocks are "pulled under."

TURN-OUT: A basic position describing the leg position in relation to the hip sockets. In a standing position, the feet can be either parallel or the toes pointed diagonally.

UNCURL: The slow, gradual straightening of the spine (vertebra by vertebra) from a rounded-back position.

187